VEGETARIAN RENAL DIET COOKBOOK FOR SENIORS

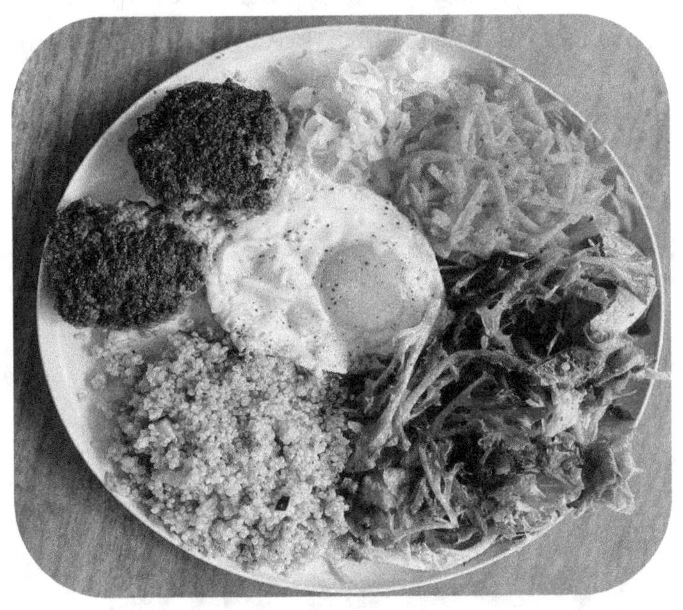

1500 DAYS OF TASTY, EASY AND NUTRITIOUS PLANT BASED RECIPES LOW IN POTASSIUM, SODIUM AND PHOSPHORUS TO MANAGE KIDNEY DISEASE, & AVOID DIALYSIS FOR A HEALTHIER LIFE.

CARLY EVELYN

SCAN TO GET MORE BOOKS BY THIS AUTHOR

IF YOU ARE STUCK, WHILE PREPARING ANY RECIPES IN THIS COOKBOOK, YOU CAN REACH THE AUTHOR AT CARLYEVLCUISINEGUIDE@GMAIL.COM FOR GUIDANCE

TABLE OF CONTENT

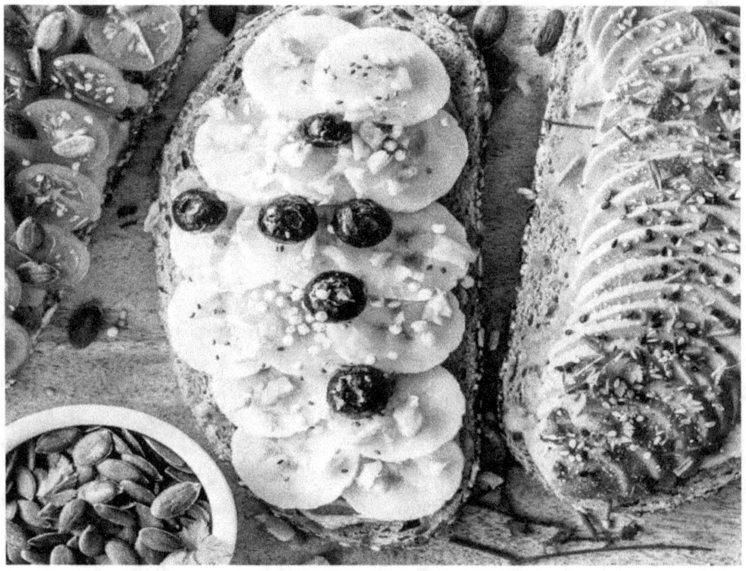

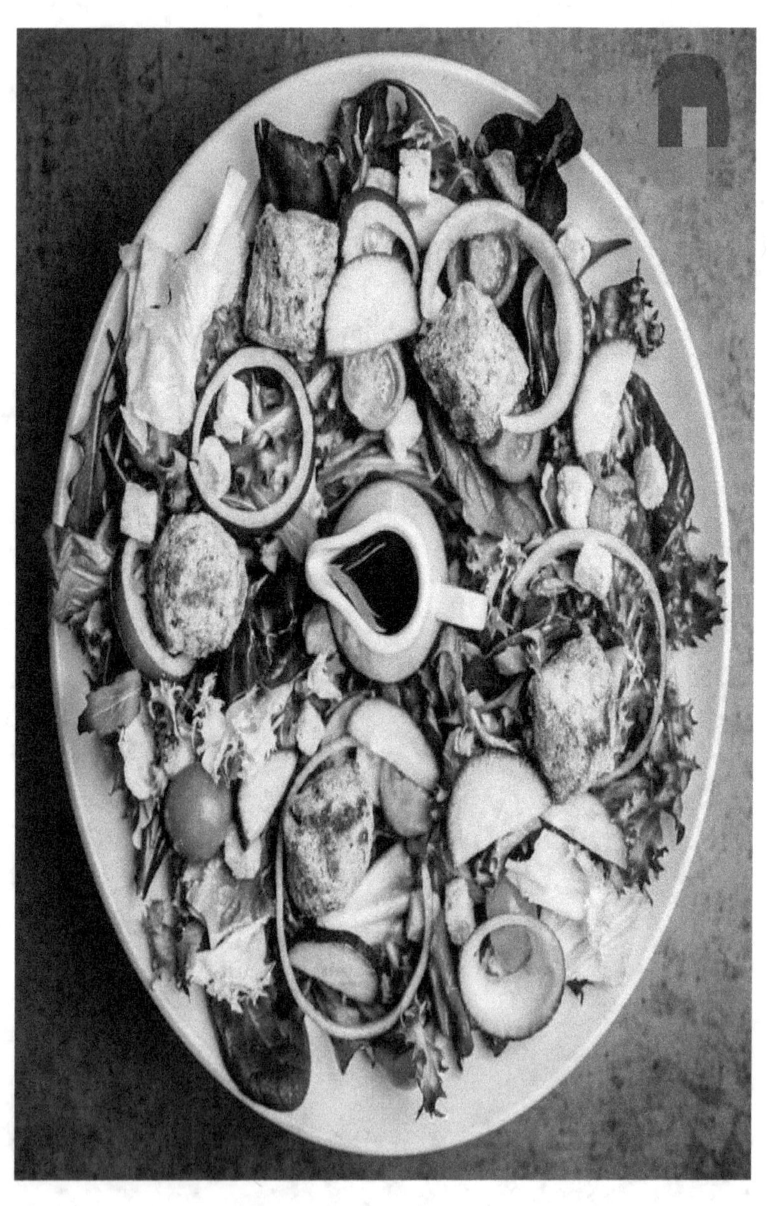

INTRODUCTION

In the setting of a small town, Emma, a single mother, faced an unexpected hurdle: kidney disease. Her diagnosis introduced uncertainty, yet Emma, driven by her steadfast love for her daughter Lily, embarked on a transformative journey to conquer this unforeseen challenge.

Refusing to let her health condition dictate her life, Emma immersed herself in research and discovered stories of individuals who had effectively managed kidney disease by adopting a plant-based, vegetarian diet. Captivated and optimistic, Emma chose to revamp her lifestyle to improve both her well-being and Lily's future.

Weekends transformed into adventures at the local farmers' market, where Emma and Lily delighted in the vivid colors of fresh, organic produce. Equipped with newfound knowledge, Emma turned their kitchen into a sanctuary for culinary experimentation.

The pair embraced the realm of vegetarian cuisine, exploring a variety of fruits, vegetables, and whole grains. Emma, now a culinary maestro, concocted meals that not only pleased their palates but also provided nourishment for her ailing kidneys. Lily, with her petite hands and infectious enthusiasm, became an essential part of the kitchen, transforming it into a space for love and learning.

Despite the obstacles, Emma's persistence yielded positive results. Regular medical check-ups showed an improvement in her kidney function. Emma's revitalized energy became contagious, and the bond between mother and daughter deepened through shared triumphs.

With the changing seasons came a positive shift in Emma's health. The kitchen, once a battleground against illness, now resonated with the laughter of a resilient mother and her spirited daughter. Together, they not only navigated the intricacies of kidney disease but also crafted a tapestry woven with love, health, and triumph against all odds.

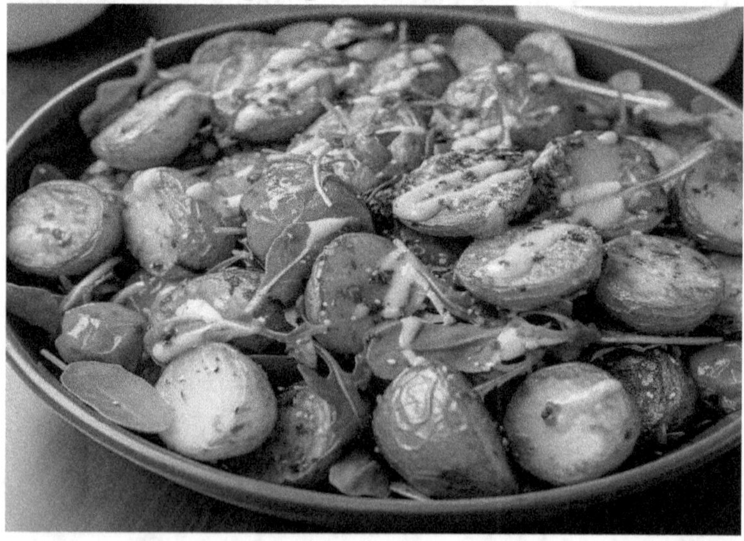

FOODS TO EAT OR AVOID ON A KIDNEY DISEASE DIET TO ACHIEVE OPTIMUM HEALTH.

A crucial role in managing kidney disease and promoting overall health is played by a specialized diet. For those maneuvering through the intricacies of kidney disease, making informed decisions about their dietary choices becomes imperative to slow down the progression of the disease and alleviate associated symptoms. Below is an extensive guide that details the foods to incorporate and avoid in a kidney disease diet for the attainment of optimal health.

RECOMMENDED FOODS:

1. Low-Potassium Fruits:
Integrate fruits with reduced potassium levels into the diet, such as apples, berries, grapes, and peaches. These fruits offer essential vitamins and antioxidants without exerting excessive stress on the kidneys.

2. Vegetables:
Opt for vegetables like cabbage, cauliflower, bell peppers, and lettuce, known for their lower potassium content. These vegetables contribute fiber, vitamins, and minerals without imposing an overwhelming burden on kidney function.

3. Lean Proteins:

Select lean protein sources, including chicken, turkey, fish, and eggs. These protein options deliver high-quality nutritional benefits without overloading the kidneys with excessive waste products.

4. Whole Grains:

Embrace whole grains like brown rice, quinoa, and whole wheat bread. These grains provide essential fiber and nutrients while maintaining lower phosphorus levels, thereby supporting kidney health.

5. Healthy Fats:

Incorporate sources of healthy fats such as olive oil, avocados, and nuts to sustain overall health. These fats are heart-friendly and offer a valuable energy source.

6. Calcium-Rich Foods:

Consume moderate amounts of calcium through foods like low-fat dairy, tofu, and leafy greens. Calcium is indispensable for bone health, and its careful incorporation is vital for those managing kidney disease.

7. Berries and Cherries:

Berries and cherries, rich in antioxidants and relatively low in potassium, make flavorful additions to meals and snacks.

8. Herbs and Spices:

Utilize herbs and spices to enhance flavor without relying on excessive salt. Fresh herbs like basil, thyme, and cilantro add taste without compromising kidney health.

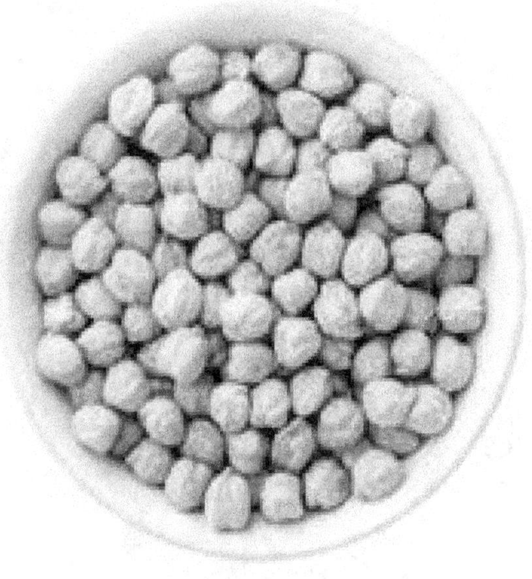

Chickpeas

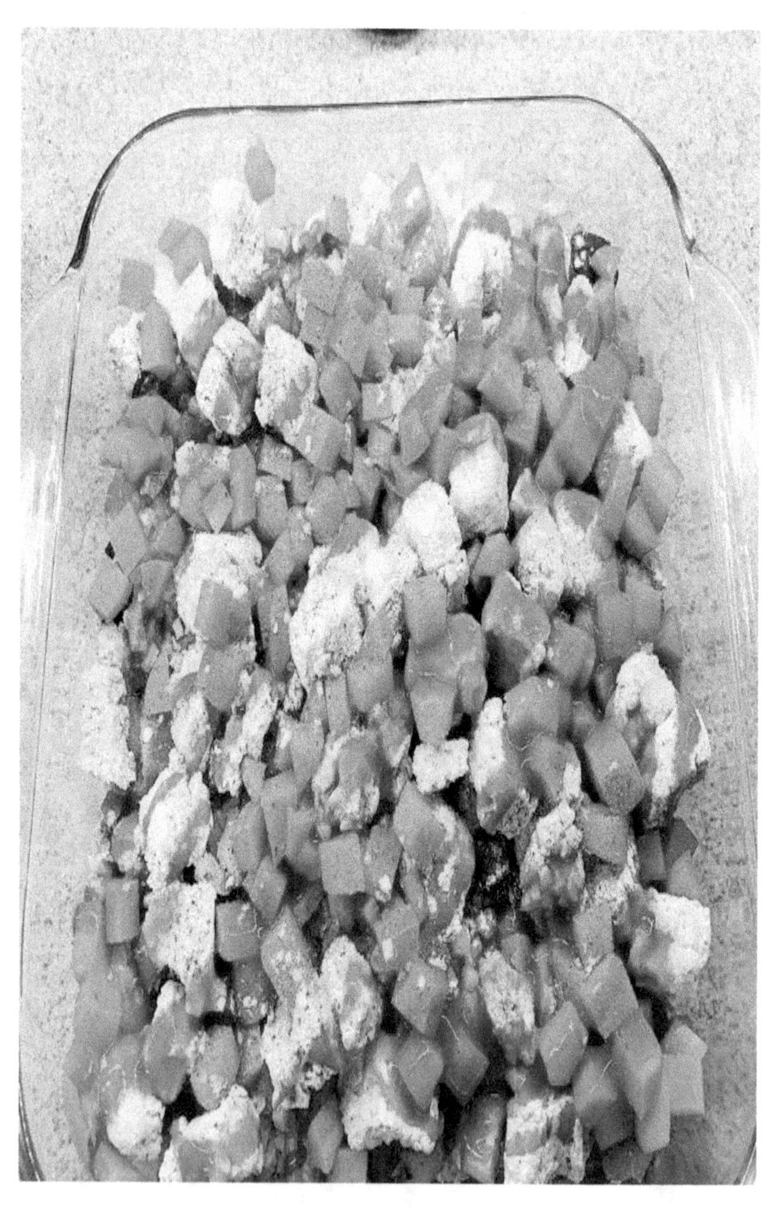

FOODS TO RESTRICT OR AVOID:

1. High-Potassium Foods:

Restrict the intake of high-potassium foods such as bananas, oranges, tomatoes, and potatoes. Elevated potassium levels can strain kidney function, leading to complications.

2. Processed Foods:

Limit processed and packaged foods, which often contain high levels of sodium, preservatives, and additives that can negatively impact kidney health.

3. Red Meat:

Reduce the consumption of red meat, as it tends to be higher in phosphorus and can contribute to the accumulation of waste products in the body.

4. Dairy Products:

Moderation in the consumption of dairy products is advised, with a preference for low-fat options, as they can be sources of phosphorus and potassium.

5. Saturated Fats:

Cut back on saturated fats present in fried foods, fatty meats, and full-fat dairy, as these fats can contribute to heart disease, a concern for individuals managing kidney disease.

<u>6. High-Sodium Foods:</u>

Manage sodium intake by steering clear of processed foods, canned soups, and fast food, as excess sodium can lead to fluid retention and high blood pressure, further compromising kidney function.

<u>7. Alcohol:</u>

Limit alcohol consumption, as it can dehydrate the body, potentially worsening complications related to kidney function.

Maintaining a well-balanced kidney disease diet involves meticulous consideration of dietary choices. Striking the right balance between essential nutrients and restricted elements is crucial for effectively managing kidney disease and promoting overall well-being.

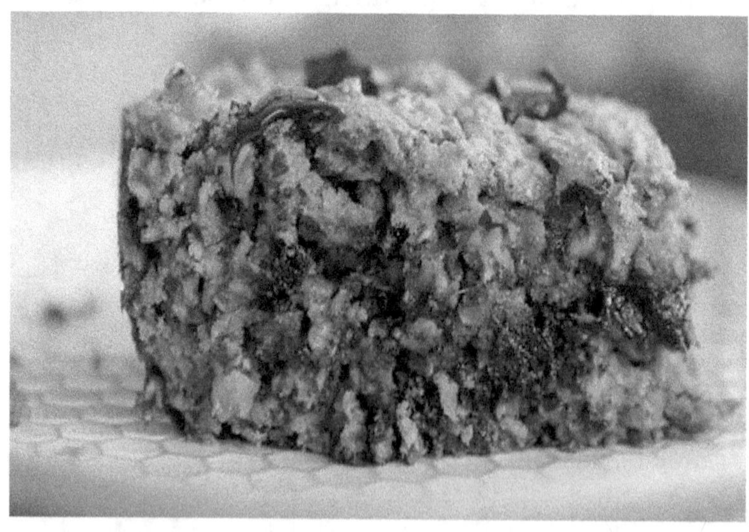

CORE BENEFITS OF FOLLOWING A KIDNEY DISEASE DIET FOR SENIORS.

Embarking on a kidney disease diet is crucial for novices seeking to effectively manage the condition and foster overall health. The following outlines key advantages of adhering to a kidney disease diet:

1. Slows Disease Progression:
A well-crafted kidney disease diet, abundant in nutrient-dense foods and minimal in substances that may strain the kidneys, plays a pivotal role in decelerating the advancement of kidney disease. This becomes indispensable for sustaining kidney function over the long term.

2. Manages Symptoms:
The kidney disease diet proves instrumental in addressing common symptoms linked to kidney disease, including fluid retention, electrolyte imbalances, and elevated blood pressure. Thoughtful dietary choices can alleviate these symptoms, leading to an improvement in overall well-being.

3. Balances Electrolytes:
Focused on achieving equilibrium among electrolytes such as potassium, phosphorus, and sodium, the diet is essential for various bodily functions. Maintaining optimal levels of these electrolytes becomes imperative

for individuals with kidney disease to avert complications.

4. Reduces Risk of Complications:
By steering clear of or moderating the intake of foods high in potassium, phosphorus, and sodium, individuals adhering to a kidney disease diet can mitigate the risk of complications like hyperkalemia, hyperphosphatemia, and hypertension—common concerns for those with kidney issues.

5. Preserves Bone Health:
The regulation of calcium, vital for individuals with kidney disease, is carefully managed within the diet to uphold bone health and forestall complications associated with irregular calcium levels.

6. Controls Blood Pressure:
The kidney disease diet places emphasis on diminishing sodium intake, contributing to the control of blood pressure. Maintaining healthy blood pressure is critical for individuals with kidney disease, as elevated levels can exacerbate kidney damage.

7. Manages Protein Intake:
Deliberate selection of protein sources is a component of the diet to regulate protein intake. This is crucial, as excessive protein can lead to the accumulation of waste

products in the blood, imposing additional stress on the kidneys.

8. Supports Heart Health:
The kidney disease diet, often aligning with heart-healthy dietary principles, bolsters cardiovascular health. Encouraging the consumption of heart-friendly foods, such as fruits, vegetables, and lean proteins, aids individuals with kidney disease in reducing the risk of cardiovascular complications.

9. Enhances Nutritional Status:
Despite constraints on specific foods, a well-structured kidney disease diet ensures individuals receive sufficient nutrients. This is fundamental for sustaining overall health and averting nutritional deficiencies.

10. Promotes Overall Well-Being:
Embracing a kidney disease diet brings about elevated energy levels, reduced symptoms, and an overall enhancement in the quality of life for individuals. Thoughtful dietary choices contribute significantly to a positive impact on both physical and mental well-being.

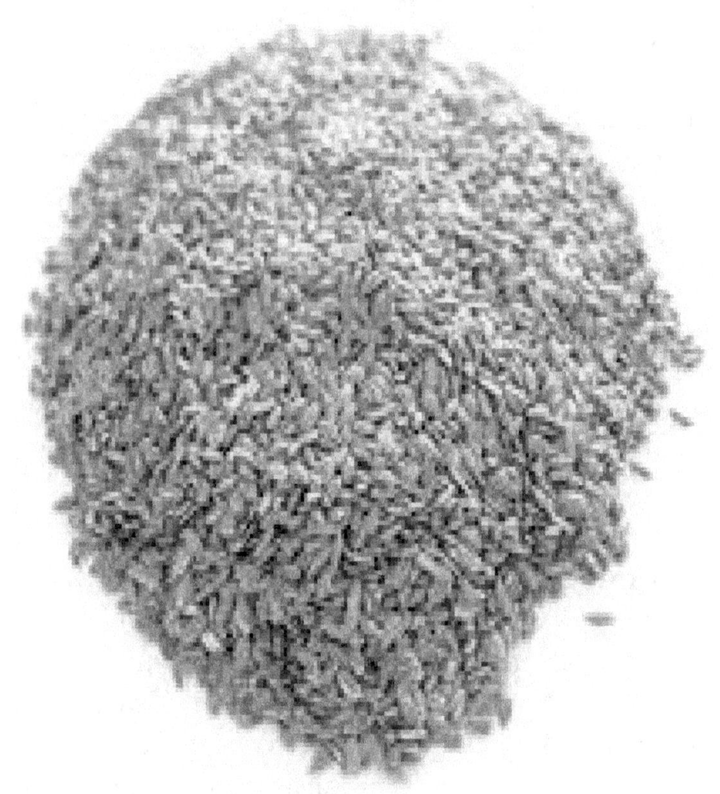

Flaxseed

HOW TO FOLLOW A KIDNEY DISEASE DIET.

Adhering to a kidney disease diet entails making specific dietary choices to effectively manage the condition and enhance overall kidney health. Here is a comprehensive guide on how to follow a kidney disease diet:

1. Consult with Healthcare Professionals:

Before implementing significant changes to your diet, seek guidance from your healthcare team, including a nephrologist and a registered dietitian. Their expertise will enable them to offer personalized advice based on your specific kidney condition, medical history, and nutritional requirements.

2. Understand Nutrient Restrictions:

Develop a clear understanding of the nutrients that require monitoring, such as potassium, phosphorus, sodium, and protein. Different stages of kidney disease may necessitate varying dietary restrictions, making it crucial to be aware of your specific requirements.

3. Educate Yourself on High and Low Nutrient Foods:

Familiarize yourself with foods that are high and low in potassium, phosphorus, sodium, and protein. This knowledge serves as the foundation for making informed food choices, ensuring that you stay within recommended limits.

4. Limit High-Potassium Foods:

Acknowledge the importance of potassium for bodily functions, but be cautious of excessive levels, which can be detrimental to those with kidney disease. Restrict intake of high-potassium foods like bananas, oranges, tomatoes, and potatoes, opting for lower-potassium alternatives such as apples, berries, and cabbage.

5. Manage Phosphorus Intake:

Exercise vigilance in monitoring phosphorus intake by reducing the consumption of processed and packaged foods, which often contain high levels of phosphorus additives. Choose whole grains, fresh fruits, and vegetables, as they are lower in phosphorus.

6. Reduce Sodium Intake:

Take steps to lower sodium intake to control blood pressure and reduce fluid retention. Steer clear of processed foods, canned soups, and fast food, and instead use herbs, spices, and other low-sodium seasonings to enhance flavor.

7. Control Protein Consumption:

Make mindful choices in managing protein intake by opting for lean protein sources like chicken, turkey, fish, and eggs. Limit the consumption of red meat and high-protein dairy products, as excessive protein can strain the kidneys.

8. Choose Heart-Healthy Fats:

Incorporate heart-healthy fats into your diet, such as olive oil, avocados, and nuts. These fats support overall health without adversely affecting kidney function.

9. Balance Fluid Intake:

Maintain a careful balance of fluid intake. While hydration is crucial, excessive fluid intake can lead to fluid retention. Adhere to the daily fluid limits recommended by your healthcare team.

10. Monitor Portion Sizes:

Exercise caution in monitoring portion sizes to avoid overconsumption of nutrients, particularly for foods higher in potassium, phosphorus, or sodium.

11. Keep a Food Diary:

Track your daily food intake to monitor adherence to dietary recommendations. A food diary also aids your healthcare team in identifying patterns and making necessary adjustments.

12. Regularly Review and Adjust:

Conduct regular reviews of your kidney disease diet with your healthcare team. Given that kidney function may change over time, adjustments to your dietary plan may be necessary.

13. Seek Support and Resources:

Engage with support groups and access educational resources related to kidney disease and nutrition. Connecting with others following a similar diet can offer valuable insights and emotional support.

14. Incorporate Lifestyle Changes:

Extend your focus beyond dietary modifications to embrace a healthy lifestyle. Engage in regular physical activity, manage stress effectively, and avoid smoking, as these factors contribute significantly to overall well-being.

By adhering to these steps and maintaining open communication with your healthcare team, you can effectively navigate and manage a kidney disease diet. The ultimate goal is to strike a balance that meets your nutritional needs while minimizing the impact on kidney function, thereby promoting overall health and enhancing your quality of life.

When adhering to a diet conducive to kidney health, it is imperative to exercise prudence during grocery shopping. Presented below are 20 nutritious items suitable for a kidney-friendly diet:

1. Fruits with Low Potassium Content:

   - Opt for apples, cranberries, and assorted berries like strawberries, blueberries, and raspberries.

2. Vegetables with Low Potassium Levels:

   - Select cabbage, cauliflower, bell peppers, lettuce, and zucchini to maintain lower potassium intake.

3. Lean Protein Sources:

   - Consider skinless chicken, turkey, and various fish options such as salmon, cod, and tilapia. Eggs are also a suitable protein choice.

4. Whole Grains:

   - Include brown rice, quinoa, oats, and whole wheat bread in your diet for a wholesome source of grains.

5. Healthy Fats:

   - Integrate olive oil, avocados, and nuts like almonds, cashews, and walnuts into your diet for heart-healthy fats.

6. Low-Phosphorus Dairy Alternatives:
   - Explore almond milk, rice milk, and cheeses with lower phosphorus content.

7. Berries and Cherries:
   - Enjoy the antioxidant-rich benefits of strawberries, blueberries, and cherries in moderation.

8. Herbs and Spices:
   - Enhance flavor with herbs such as basil, thyme, cilantro, and garlic, minimizing the need for excessive salt.

9. Low-Sodium Condiments:
   - Choose condiments wisely by opting for mustard, vinegar, lemon juice, and low-sodium soy sauce.

10. Low-Potassium Pasta and Rice:
   - Include white rice and pasta made from refined flour in your diet, ensuring lower potassium content.

11. Low-Phosphorus Snacks:
   - Enjoy snacks like popcorn, rice cakes, and unsalted pretzels with reduced phosphorus levels.

12. Low-Potassium Beverages:

- Stay hydrated with water, herbal teas without added potassium, and homemade lemonade using controlled potassium ingredients.

13. Low-Phosphorus Grains:

- Include barley, bulgur, and couscous for their lower phosphorus content.

14. Calcium-Rich Foods (in moderation):

- Consume low-phosphorus dairy, tofu, and kale to meet calcium needs while being mindful of phosphorus levels.

15. Low-Potassium Canned Fruits (in juice, not syrup):

- When opting for canned fruits, choose peaches and pears in juice rather than syrup.

16. Low-Sodium Broths:

- Incorporate vegetable broth and low-sodium chicken broth into your cooking for flavor without excessive sodium.

17. Low-Phosphorus Desserts:

- Indulge in desserts like sorbet and gelatin with reduced phosphorus content.

<u>**18. Fresh Vegetables (in moderation):**</u>
   - Include fresh vegetables like carrots, green beans, and cucumbers in measured amounts.

<u>**19. Low-Potassium Cooking Ingredients:**</u>
   - Use cooking ingredients such as cornstarch, flour, and baking powder, which are lower in potassium.

<u>**20. Low-Sodium Canned Beans:**</u>
   - Choose canned beans like kidney beans and black beans, rinsing them to reduce potassium levels.

It's essential to note that individual dietary requirements may differ based on the stage of kidney disease and other health considerations. Seeking guidance from healthcare professionals or registered dietitians specializing in kidney health ensures the creation of a tailored and effective meal plan aligned with specific needs.

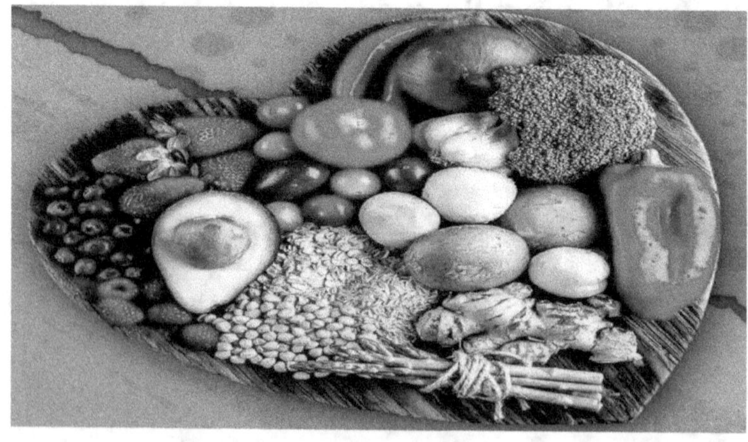

COMPLICATIONS OF KIDNEY DISEASE, IF THE RIGHT DIET ISN'T ADOPTED.

Neglecting to adopt an appropriate diet while managing kidney disease can result in a variety of complications, given the pivotal role of kidneys in maintaining overall health. The following outlines potential complications linked to kidney disease when a suitable diet is not implemented:

1. Advancement of Kidney Disease:
  - In the absence of dietary adjustments, the kidneys may continue to deteriorate, leading to a gradual decline in kidney function and the progression of kidney disease to more severe stages.

2. Imbalances in Fluid and Electrolytes:
  - The kidneys are responsible for regulating the body's fluid and electrolyte balance. Without adhering to a proper diet, imbalances in sodium, potassium, and phosphorus levels may occur, resulting in complications like fluid retention (edema), elevated potassium (hyperkalemia), and elevated phosphorus (hyperphosphatemia).

3. Elevated Blood Pressure:
  - Kidney disease is both a common cause and consequence of high blood pressure. Without dietary interventions to manage sodium intake and control

fluid balance, blood pressure may remain elevated, contributing to further kidney damage and cardiovascular complications.

4. Cardiovascular Challenges:
- Kidney disease is closely associated with an increased risk of cardiovascular issues. Insufficient dietary control can exacerbate this risk, as imbalances in fluids, electrolytes, and blood pressure may contribute to heart-related complications, including heart failure and heart attacks.

5. Disorders in Bone and Minerals:
- Kidneys play a pivotal role in maintaining bone health by regulating calcium and phosphorus levels. In kidney disease, imbalances in these minerals can occur, leading to conditions such as renal osteodystrophy. Without adequate dietary management, bone density may decrease, increasing the likelihood of fractures.

6. Development or Worsening of Anemia:
- Erythropoietin, a hormone produced by healthy kidneys, stimulates red blood cell production. Impaired erythropoietin production in kidney disease can lead to anemia. Without dietary adjustments to support iron absorption and maintain adequate vitamin B12 levels, anemia can worsen, causing fatigue and weakness.

7. Uremia Onset:

- Uremia, characterized by the accumulation of waste products and toxins in the blood due to impaired kidney function, may progress without dietary restrictions on protein intake and other waste-producing substances. This progression can result in symptoms such as nausea, fatigue, and confusion.

8. Compromised Immune Function:

- Kidneys contribute to immune function, and in advanced kidney disease, the immune system may be compromised. Without a supportive diet, individuals may become more susceptible to infections.

9. Nutritional Deficiencies:

- Kidney disease can impact the body's ability to process and eliminate certain nutrients. In the absence of careful dietary planning, individuals may experience nutritional deficiencies, affecting overall health and well-being.

10. Potential Hospitalization and Interventions:

- Uncontrolled kidney disease can lead to complications that may necessitate hospitalization and medical interventions, including dialysis or kidney transplantation.

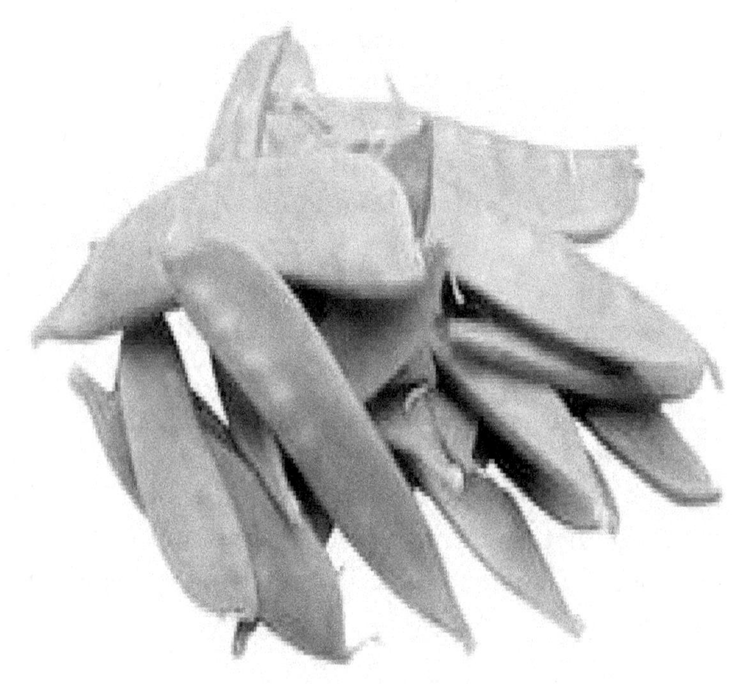

Snow Peas

MEAL PLANNING FOR KIDNEY DISEASE DIET, HIGHLIGHTING IT'S BENEFITS FOR PROPER MANAGEMENT.

Effective management of kidney disease hinges on the critical element of meal planning to support kidney health and overall well-being. Below is an elucidation of the meal planning process for kidney disease, accompanied by its advantages:

Meal Planning for Kidney Disease:

1. Consultation with Healthcare Professionals:
  - Begin by engaging with healthcare experts, including nephrologists and registered dietitians specialized in renal nutrition. They will evaluate your specific condition, kidney function, and nutritional requirements.

2. Understanding Dietary Restrictions:
  - Attain a comprehensive grasp of dietary restrictions, encompassing constraints on sodium, potassium, phosphorus, and protein intake. Distinct stages of kidney disease may necessitate varying degrees of limitation.

3. Balancing Nutrients:
  - Devise meal plans that ensure an equilibrium of essential nutrients while adhering to prescribed

restrictions. This involves the careful management of protein, control of phosphorus and potassium levels, and monitoring of fluid intake.

4. Emphasis on High-Quality Proteins:
- Select high-quality protein sources, such as lean meats, poultry, fish, eggs, and plant-based proteins like tofu and legumes. Adequate protein intake is pivotal for preserving muscle mass without imposing excessive strain on the kidneys.

5. Portion Control:
- Implement portion control strategies to prevent the overconsumption of nutrients requiring moderation, such as phosphorus and potassium. Regulating portion sizes assists in maintaining a harmonious balance of nutrients.

6. Low-Sodium Cooking and Seasoning:
- Employ cooking methods that mitigate the necessity for excessive salt. Opt for herbs, spices, and other low-sodium seasonings to enhance flavor without compromising kidney health.

7. Incorporating Low-Potassium Fruits and Vegetables:
- Infuse meal plans with low-potassium fruits and vegetables, including apples, berries, cabbage, cauliflower, and lettuce. These choices provide

essential vitamins and minerals without elevating potassium levels.

8. Whole Grains and Low-Phosphorus Choices:
- Opt for whole grains like brown rice and quinoa, and choose alternatives low in phosphorus. This ensures a rich source of fiber and nutrients without escalating phosphorus intake.

9. Monitoring Fluid Intake:
- Plan meals to strike a balance in fluid intake, as excessive fluid can strain the kidneys. Adhere to recommended daily fluid limits as advised by healthcare professionals.

10. Regular Meal Timing:
- Establish consistent meal times to foster regularity in nutrient intake. This aids in managing blood sugar levels and supporting overall health.

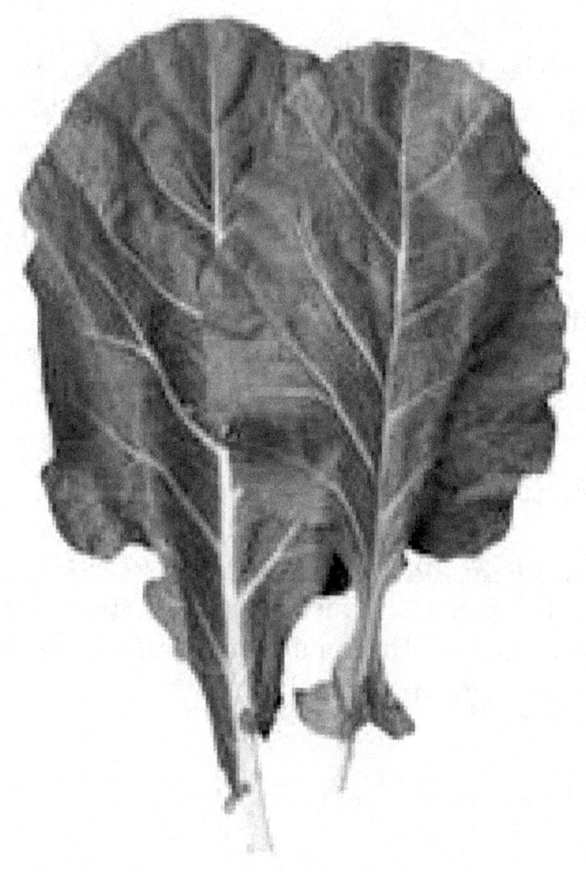

Collard Greens

BENEFITS OF MEAL PLANNING FOR KIDNEY DISEASE:

1. Disease Management:
- Proficient meal planning plays a pivotal role in effectively managing kidney disease, slowing down its progression and preserving kidney function over time.

2. Symptom Control:
- Well-constructed meal plans assist in managing common symptoms associated with kidney disease, including fluid retention, electrolyte imbalances, and high blood pressure.

3. Prevention of Complications:
- Adherence to a kidney-friendly diet helps thwart complications such as hyperkalemia, hyperphosphatemia, and hypertension, mitigating the risk of additional health issues.

4. Bone Health Preservation:
- Through meticulous management of calcium and phosphorus levels, the diet contributes to the preservation of bone health, diminishing the risk of bone disorders linked to kidney disease.

5. Controlled Blood Pressure:
- Meal plans emphasizing low-sodium choices contribute to maintaining controlled blood pressure,

thereby reducing the strain on the kidneys and lessening cardiovascular risks.

6. Balanced Nutrition:

- Thoughtful meal planning ensures individuals receive a well-rounded nutritional profile despite dietary restrictions, averting nutritional deficiencies and supporting overall health.

7. Enhanced Quality of Life:

- Adhering to a well-structured meal plan customized for kidney disease fosters an improved quality of life, enabling individuals to relish a variety of foods while effectively managing their condition.

8. Individualized Approach:

- Meal planning is individualized based on specific needs, rendering it a tailored and effective strategy for managing kidney disease.

9. Empowerment and Engagement:

- Actively participating in meal planning empowers individuals and engages them in their health management, fostering a proactive approach to nutrition and overall well-being.

10. Collaboration with Healthcare Professionals:

- Meal planning facilitates ongoing collaboration with healthcare professionals, ensuring necessary adjustments are made based on changes in kidney function and overall health.

Meal planning is an indispensable cornerstone in the effective management of kidney disease. It not only addresses specific dietary needs but also promotes overall health, symptom control, and an improved quality of life for individuals navigating the complexities of kidney disease.

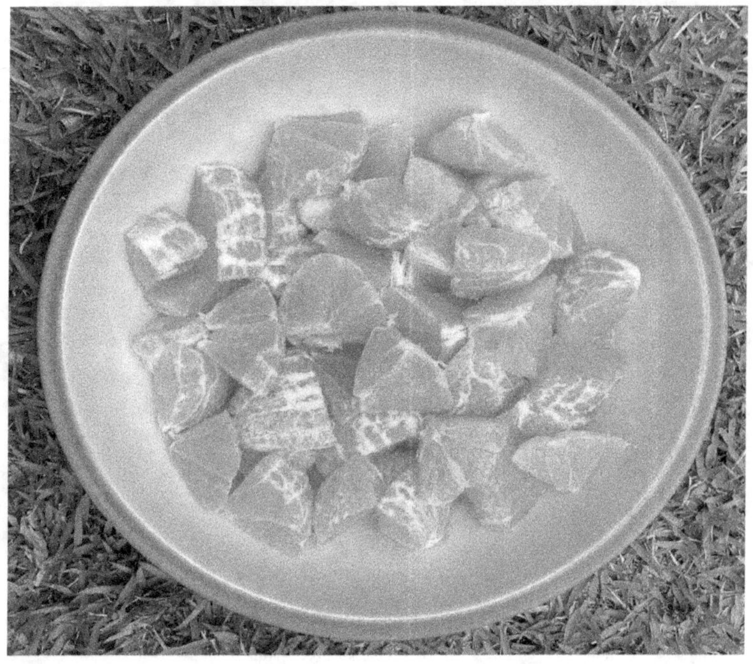

Spaghetti Squash

SERIAL 14-DAY SAMPLE KIDNEY DISEASE MEAL PLAN.

Creating a sample meal plan for kidney disease involves thoughtful consideration of nutrient restrictions and individual preferences. Below is a 14-day sample meal plan, emphasizing low-sodium, low-potassium, and controlled protein intake.

Day 1:

- Breakfast:
  - Oatmeal with sliced apples (low-potassium fruit)
  - Scrambled eggs

- Lunch:
  - Grilled chicken breast (portion-controlled)
  - Quinoa salad with cucumber and cherry tomatoes
  - Steamed green beans

- Snack:
  - Greek yogurt (low-phosphorus) with a drizzle of honey
  - Rice cakes

- Dinner:
  - Baked salmon (portion-controlled)
  - Mashed sweet potatoes
  - Steamed broccoli

Day 2:

- **Breakfast:**
  - Whole grain toast with avocado (healthy fats)
  - Fresh berries (low-potassium)

- **Lunch:**
  - Turkey and vegetable wrap with whole grain tortilla
  - Carrot sticks

- **Snack:**
  - Almonds (portion-controlled)
  - Apple slices

- **Dinner:**
  - Lentil soup
  - Brown rice
  - Grilled asparagus

Day 3:

- **Breakfast:**
  - Smoothie with spinach, banana, and almond milk (low-phosphorus)

- **Lunch:**
  - Tofu stir-fry with mixed vegetables
  - Quinoa

- **Snack:**
  - Cottage cheese (low-phosphorus) with pineapple

- **Dinner:**
  - Baked chicken thighs (portion-controlled)
  - Steamed cauliflower
  - Wild rice

Day 4:

- **Breakfast:**
  - Low-phosphorus cereal with almond milk
  - Peach slices

- **Lunch:**
  - Shrimp and vegetable kebabs
  - Couscous

- **Snack:**
  - Rice crackers with hummus

- **Dinner:**
  - Beef stew with low-sodium broth
  - Quinoa
  - Steamed green beans

Day 5:

- Breakfast:
 - Whole grain waffle with strawberries (low-potassium)
 - Scrambled eggs

- Lunch:
 - Grilled fish tacos with cabbage slaw
 - Black beans (rinsed to reduce potassium)

- Snack:
 - Celery sticks with peanut butter (portion-controlled)

- Dinner:
 - Eggplant lasagna with ground turkey
 - Mixed salad with vinaigrette dressing

Day 6:

- Breakfast:
 - Smoothie with kale, banana, and almond milk (low-phosphorus)

- Lunch:
 - Chicken and vegetable curry with basmati rice

- Snack:
  - Greek yogurt (low-phosphorus) with a sprinkle of chia seeds

- Dinner:
  - Baked cod fillets (portion-controlled)
  - Quinoa salad with cherry tomatoes and cucumber

Day 7:

- Breakfast:
  - Low-phosphorus granola with almond milk
  - Fresh orange slices

- Lunch:
  - Turkey and avocado wrap with whole grain tortilla
  - Roasted sweet potato wedges

- Snack:
  - Apple slices with a small amount of cheese (low-phosphorus)

- Dinner:
  - Grilled chicken breast (portion-controlled)
  - Brown rice
  - Steamed broccoli and carrots

Day 8:

- Breakfast:
  - Whole grain toast with almond butter
  - Sliced kiwi (low-potassium)

- Lunch:
  - Vegetable and chickpea salad
  - Quinoa

- Snack:
  - Cottage cheese (low-phosphorus) with sliced peaches

- Dinner:
  - Grilled shrimp skewers
  - Brown rice
  - Steamed asparagus

Day 9:

- Breakfast:
  - Scrambled eggs with diced tomatoes and spinach
  - Whole grain English muffin

- Lunch:
  - Lentil and vegetable soup
  - Whole wheat roll

- **Snack:**
  - Mixed nuts (portion-controlled)
  - Fresh pear slices

- **Dinner:**
  - Baked chicken thighs (portion-controlled)
  - Quinoa salad with cucumber and cherry tomatoes

Day 10:

- **Breakfast:**
  - Smoothie with mixed berries (low-potassium), spinach, and almond milk

- **Lunch:**
  - Turkey and vegetable stir-fry with brown rice
  - Steamed broccoli

- **Snack:**
  - Rice cakes with hummus
  - Apple slices

- **Dinner:**
  - Grilled fish fillets (portion-controlled)
  - Couscous
  - Roasted Brussels sprouts

Day 11:

- Breakfast:
  - Low-phosphorus yogurt parfait with granola and strawberries
  - Hard-boiled eggs

- Lunch:
  - Chicken Caesar salad with a light dressing
  - Whole grain croutons

- Snack:
  - Celery sticks with peanut butter (portion-controlled)

- Dinner:
  - Eggplant and chickpea curry with basmati rice
  - Steamed green beans

Day 12:

- Breakfast:
  - Whole grain waffle with banana slices and a drizzle of honey
  - Scrambled eggs

- Lunch:
  - Grilled vegetable and feta cheese wrap with whole grain tortilla
  - Carrot sticks

- Snack:
  - Greek yogurt (low-phosphorus) with a sprinkle of chia seeds

- Dinner:
  - Baked cod fillets (portion-controlled)
  - Quinoa
  - Steamed asparagus

Day 13:

- Breakfast:
  - Low-phosphorus cereal with almond milk
  - Fresh mango slices (low-potassium)

- Lunch:
  - Shrimp and vegetable stir-fry with brown rice
  - Snow peas

- Snack:
  - Rice crackers with guacamole

- Dinner:
  - Turkey meatballs with whole wheat spaghetti
  - Tomato and basil sauce

- **Breakfast:**
  - Smoothie with kale, pineapple, and coconut water
  - Whole grain toast with avocado

- **Lunch:**
  - Quinoa salad with black beans, corn, and tomatoes
  - Sliced oranges

- **Snack:**
  - Cottage cheese (low-phosphorus) with mixed berries

- **Dinner:**
  - Grilled chicken breast (portion-controlled)
  - Brown rice
  - Roasted sweet potato wedges

Don't forget to adapt the meal plan to individual needs, preferences,

10 KIDNEY DISEASE BREAKFAST RECIPES

Ten kidney-friendly breakfast recipes with ingredients, preparation methods, quantity measurements, nutritional values, and cooking duration.

1. Berry Oatmeal

- Ingredients:
- 1/2 cup of rolled oats
- 1 cup of water
- 1/2 cup of mixed berries (blueberries, strawberries)
- 1 tablespoon chia seeds
- 1 tablespoon honey

- Preparation:
1. Boil 1 cup of water and add rolled oats.
2. Cook for 5-7 minutes until the oats are soft.
3. Top with mixed berries, chia seeds, and honey.

- Nutritional Value:
- Calories: 250
- Protein: 7g
- Fiber: 8g
- Potassium: 200mg

- Cooking Duration :10 minutes

2. Spinach Scrambled Eggs

- Ingredients:
  - 2 large eggs
  - 1 cup of fresh spinach, chopped
  - 1 tablespoon olive oil
  - Salt and pepper to taste

- Preparation:
  1. Heat 1 tablespoon of olive oil in a pan and sauté spinach until wilted.
  2. Whisk eggs, pour into the pan, and scramble.
  3. Season with salt and pepper.

- Nutritional Value:
  - Calories: 220
  - Protein: 15g
  - Iron: 2mg

- Cooking Duration :8 minutes

3. Avocado Toast

- Ingredients:
  - 2 slices whole-grain bread
  - 1/2 ripe avocado, mashed
  - 1 teaspoon lemon juice
  - Pinch of salt

- Preparation:
  1. Toast the slices of bread.
  2. Mix mashed avocado with lemon juice and salt.
  3. Spread avocado on the toast.

- Nutritional Value:
  - Calories: 230
  - Fiber: 8g
  - Potassium: 350mg

- Cooking Duration :5 minutes

4. Greek Yogurt Parfait

- Ingredients:
  - 1 cup of Greek yogurt (low-phosphorus)
  - 1/4 cup of granola
  - 1/2 cup of mixed berries
  - 1 tablespoon honey

- **Preparation:**
   1. Layer Greek yogurt, granola, and berries.
   2. Drizzle with honey.

- **Nutritional Value:**
   - Calories: 300
   - Protein: 20g
   - Calcium: 200mg

- **Cooking Duration :**5 minutes

5. Nutty Berry Smoothie Bowl

- **Ingredients:**
   - 1/2 cup of frozen mixed berries
   - 1/2 banana
   - 1/2 cup of low-phosphorus yogurt
   - 1 tablespoon almond butter
   - 1 tablespoon chia seeds

- **Preparation:**
   1. Blend berries, banana, and yogurt until smooth.
   2. Pour into a bowl and top with almond butter and chia seeds.

- **Nutritional Value:**
   - Calories: 280
   - Protein: 12g
   - Fiber: 10g

- Cooking Duration :5 minutes

6. Cottage Cheese and Pineapple Bowl

- Ingredients:
  - 1/2 cup of low-phosphorus cottage cheese
  - 1/2 cup of fresh pineapple, diced
  - 1 tablespoon shredded coconut

- Preparation:
  1. Mix cottage cheese and diced pineapple.
  2. Sprinkle with shredded coconut.

- Nutritional Value:
  - Calories: 180
  - Protein: 15g
  - Calcium: 100mg

- Cooking Duration :5 minutes

7. Quinoa Breakfast Bowl

- Ingredients:
  - 1/2 cup of cooked quinoa
  - 1/4 cup of almond milk
  - 1/4 cup of sliced strawberries
  - 1 tablespoon chopped nuts (walnuts, almonds)

- Preparation:
 1. Warm cooked quinoa with almond milk.
 2. Top with sliced strawberries and chopped nuts.

- Nutritional Value:
 - Calories: 220
 - Protein: 7g
 - Fiber: 5g

- Cooking Duration :7 minutes

8. Banana Pancakes

- Ingredients:
 - 1 ripe banana
 - 2 eggs
 - 1/4 teaspoon vanilla extract
 - 1/4 teaspoon cinnamon

- Preparation:
 1. Mash banana, whisk in eggs, vanilla, and cinnamon.
 2. Pour onto a hot griddle, cook until edges set, and flip.

- Nutritional Value:
 - Calories: 250
 - Protein: 12g
 - Potassium: 400mg

- **Cooking Duration :**10 minutes

9. Almond Butter Rice Cake

- **Ingredients:**
  - 2 rice cakes
  - 2 tablespoons almond butter
  - 1/2 banana, sliced

- **Preparation:**
  1. Spread almond butter on rice cakes.
  2. Top with sliced banana.

- **Nutritional Value:**
  - Calories: 280
  - Protein: 7g
  - Fiber: 4g

- **Cooking Duration :**3 minutes

10. Spinach and Feta Omelet

- **Ingredients:**
  - 3 eggs
  - 1 cup of fresh spinach, chopped
  - 2 tablespoons feta cheese, crumbled
  - Salt and pepper to taste

- Preparation:
1. Whisk eggs and pour into a hot, greased pan.
2. Add spinach, feta, salt, and pepper. Fold when set.

- Nutritional Value:
- Calories: 280
- Protein: 20g
- Iron: 3mg

- Cooking Duration :8 minutes

Note: Nutritional values are approximate and may vary based on specific brands and quantities used. Adjust portion sizes according to your dietary needs

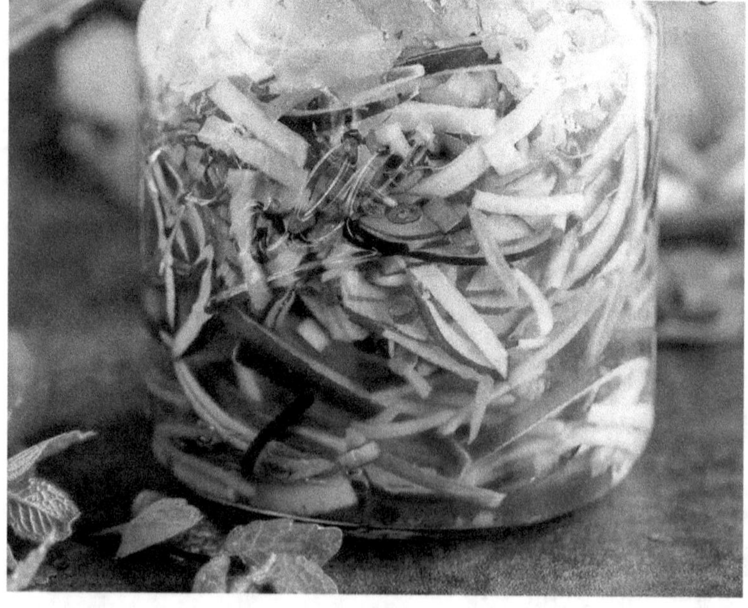

10 KIDNEY DISEASE LUNCH RECIPES

Ten lunch recipes tailored to kidney-friendly guidelines, complete with ingredients, preparation techniques, quantities, nutritional content, and cooking durations:

1. Grilled Lemon Herb Chicken Salad

Ingredients:
- 4 boneless, skinless chicken breasts
- 2 tablespoons olive oil
- 1 teaspoon dried oregano
- 1 teaspoon dried thyme
- 1 teaspoon garlic powder
- Juice of 1 lemon
- Salt and pepper to taste
- 8 cup of mixed salad greens

Preparation:
1. Preheat the grill to medium-high heat.
2. Combine olive oil, oregano, thyme, garlic powder, lemon juice, salt, and pepper in a bowl.
3. Brush the chicken breasts with the mixture and grill for 6-8 minutes per side.
4. Slice the chicken and serve over a bed of mixed salad greens.

Nutritional Value:

- Calories: 300
- Protein: 35g
- Sodium: 80mg
- Phosphorus: 200mg
- Potassium: 450mg

Cooking Duration :20 minutes

2. Quinoa and Vegetable Stir-Fry

Ingredients:
- 1 cup of quinoa
- 2 cup of water
- 2 tablespoons low-sodium soy sauce
- 1 tablespoon olive oil
- 1 cup of broccoli florets
- 1 bell pepper, thinly sliced
- 1 cup of snap peas
- 2 cloves garlic, minced

Preparation:

1. Rinse the quinoa and cook it in water according to package instructions.

2. Heat olive oil in a pan, add garlic, and stir-fry vegetables until tender.

3. Add cooked quinoa and soy sauce, tossing until well combined.

Nutritional Value:

- Calories: 320
- Protein: 12g
- Sodium: 150mg
- Phosphorus: 180mg
- Potassium: 300mg

Cooking Duration :25 minutes

3. Turkey and Vegetable Skewers

Ingredients:

- 1 pound turkey breast, cubed
- 1 zucchini, sliced
- 1 red onion, chunked
- 1 bell pepper, chunked
- 2 tablespoons olive oil
- 1 teaspoon dried rosemary
- 1 teaspoon lemon zest
- Salt and pepper to taste

Preparation:
1. Preheat the grill or oven broiler.
2. Mix turkey, vegetables, olive oil, rosemary, lemon zest, salt, and pepper in a bowl.
3. Thread turkey and vegetables onto skewers and grill for 10-12 minutes, turning occasionally.

Nutritional Value:
- Calories: 250
- Protein: 30g
- Sodium: 70mg
- Phosphorus: 220mg
- Potassium: 380mg

Cooking Duration :15 minutes

4. Lentil and Vegetable Soup

Ingredients:
- 1 cup of dried green lentils, rinsed
- 6 cup of low-sodium vegetable broth
- 1 onion, diced
- 2 carrots, sliced
- 2 celery stalks, chopped
- 2 cloves garlic, minced
- 1 teaspoon dried thyme
- 1 bay leaf
- Salt and pepper to taste

Preparation:

1. In a large pot, combine lentils, broth, onion, carrots, celery, garlic, thyme, bay leaf, salt, and pepper.
2. Bring to a boil, then reduce heat and simmer for 25-30 minutes until lentils are tender.

Nutritional Value:

- Calories: 220
- Protein: 15g
- Sodium: 100mg
- Phosphorus: 180mg
- Potassium: 400mg

Cooking Duration :35 minutes

5. Baked Salmon with Dill Sauce

Ingredients:

- 4 salmon fillets
- 2 tablespoons olive oil
- 1 lemon, sliced
- 1 teaspoon dried dill
- Salt and pepper to taste

Preparation:

1. Preheat the oven to 400°F (200°C).
2. Place salmon fillets on a baking sheet, drizzle with olive oil, sprinkle with dried dill, salt, and pepper.

3. Top each fillet with lemon slices and bake for 15-20 minutes.

Nutritional Value:
- Calories: 280
- Protein: 30g
- Sodium: 80mg
- Phosphorus: 250mg
- Potassium: 350mg

Cooking Duration :20 minutes

6. Eggplant and Tomato Stacks

Ingredients:
- 2 large eggplants, sliced
- 2 large tomatoes, sliced
- 1 cup of low-fat mozzarella, shredded
- 2 tablespoons olive oil
- 1 teaspoon dried basil
- Salt and pepper to taste

Preparation:

1. Preheat the oven to 375°F (190°C).
2. Brush eggplant slices with olive oil, sprinkle with salt and pepper.
3. In a baking dish, layer eggplant, tomato, and mozzarella. Repeat.
4. Sprinkle dried basil on top and bake for 25-30 minutes.

Nutritional Value:

- Calories: 180
- Protein: 8g
- Sodium: 90mg
- Phosphorus: 150mg
- Potassium: 300mg

Cooking Duration :30 minutes

7. Shrimp and Asparagus Stir-Fry

Ingredients:

- 1 pound shrimp, peeled and deveined
- 1 bunch asparagus, trimmed and cut into 2-inch pieces
- 2 tablespoons low-sodium soy sauce
- 1 tablespoon sesame oil
- 1 tablespoon ginger, minced
- 2 cloves garlic, minced

Preparation:

1. In a wok or large skillet, heat sesame oil and sauté garlic and ginger.
2. Add shrimp and cook until pink, then add asparagus and soy sauce.
3. Stir-fry until asparagus is tender-crisp.

Nutritional Value:

- Calories: 220
- Protein: 25g
- Sodium: 200mg
- Phosphorus: 200mg
- Potassium: 400mg

Cooking Duration :15 minutes

8. Spinach and Mushroom Frittata

Ingredients:

- 6 large eggs
- 1 cup of spinach, chopped
- 1 cup of mushrooms, sliced
- 1/2 cup of low-fat feta cheese, crumbled
- 1 tablespoon olive oil
- Salt and pepper to taste

Preparation:

1. Preheat the oven to 350°F (175°C).

2. In an oven-safe skillet, sauté mushrooms and spinach in olive oil until wilted.

3. In a bowl, beat eggs, season with salt and pepper, and pour over vegetables.

4. Sprinkle feta on top and bake for 15-20 minutes until set.

Nutritional Value:

- Calories: 200
- Protein: 15g
- Sodium: 250mg
- Phosphorus: 200mg
- Potassium: 350mg

Cooking Duration :20 minutes

9. Chicken and Vegetable Stir-Fry with Brown Rice

Ingredients:

- 1-pound boneless, skinless chicken breasts, thinly sliced
- 2 cup of broccoli florets
- 1 red bell pepper, sliced
- 1 cup of snow peas
- 2 tablespoons low-sodium soy sauce
- 1 tablespoon rice vinegar
- 1 tablespoon canola oil
- 2 cup of cooked brown rice

Preparation:

1. In a wok or large skillet, heat canola oil and stir-fry chicken until cooked.

2. Add vegetables, soy sauce, and rice vinegar, stir-fry until vegetables are tender.

3. Serve over cooked brown rice.

Nutritional Value:

- Calories: 400
- Protein: 35g
- Sodium: 300mg
- Phosphorus: 250mg
- Potassium: 500mg

Cooking Duration :25 minutes

10. Greek Salad with Grilled Chicken

Ingredients:

- 2 boneless, skinless chicken breasts
- 1 cucumber, diced
- 1 cup of cherry tomatoes, halved
- 1/2 cup of Kalamata olives, pitted and sliced
- 1/2 cup of feta cheese, crumbled
- 2 tablespoons olive oil
- 1 teaspoon dried oregano
- Salt and pepper to taste

Preparation:

1. Season chicken breasts with olive oil, oregano, salt, and pepper. Grill until cooked through.
2. Slice grilled chicken and arrange on a plate with cucumber, tomatoes, olives, and feta.
3. Drizzle with extra olive oil and sprinkle with oregano.

Nutritional Value:

- Calories: 380
- Protein: 30g
- Sodium:400mg
- Phosphorus: 300mg
- Potassium: 450mg

Cooking Duration :15 minutes

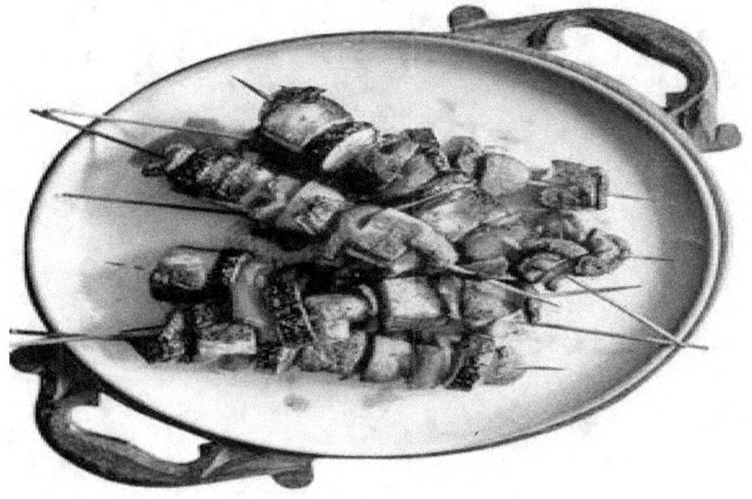

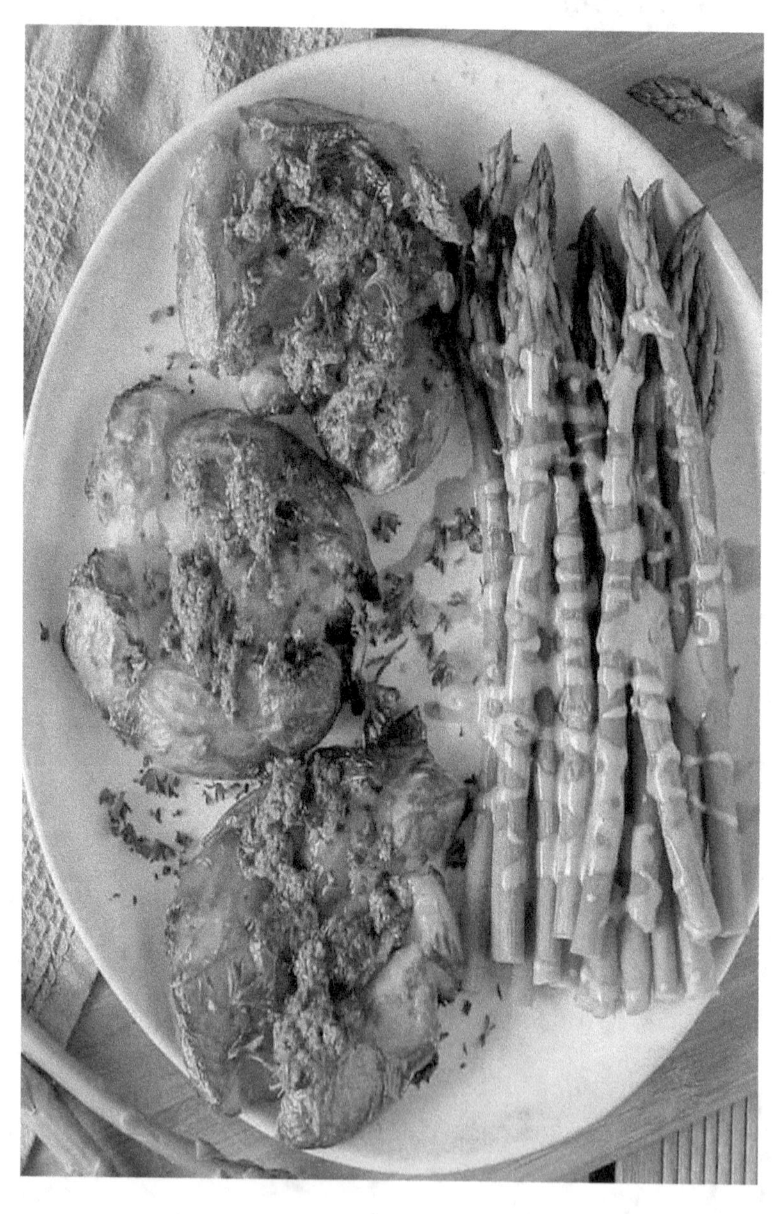

Ten kidney-friendly dinner recipes with detailed ingredients, preparation methods, quantities, nutritional information, and cooking times:

1. Herb-Crusted Baked Cod

Ingredients:
- 4 cod fillets (6 oz each)
- 2 tablespoons olive oil
- 1 tablespoon fresh parsley, chopped
- 1 teaspoon dried thyme
- 1 teaspoon garlic powder
- Salt and pepper to taste
- 1 lemon, sliced

Preparation:
1. Preheat the oven to 400°F (200°C).
2. Place the cod fillets on a baking sheet.
3. Combine olive oil, parsley, thyme, garlic powder, salt, and pepper.
4. Brush the mixture over cod fillets and top with lemon slices.
5. Bake for 15-20 minutes or until the fish flakes easily.

Nutritional Value:
- Calories: 250
- Protein: 30g

- Sodium: 100mg
- Phosphorus: 200mg
- Potassium: 400mg

Cooking Duration :20 minutes

2. Cauliflower and Chickpea Curry

Ingredients:
- 1 cauliflower, cut into florets
- 1 can (15 oz) chickpeas, drained
- 1 onion, diced
- 2 tomatoes, diced
- 1 can (14 oz) coconut milk
- 2 tablespoons curry powder
- 1 teaspoon ground turmeric
- Salt and pepper to taste
- 2 tablespoons olive oil

Preparation:
1. In a pan, sauté the onion in olive oil until translucent.
2. Add cauliflower, chickpeas, tomatoes, curry powder, turmeric, salt, and pepper.
3. Pour in coconut milk and simmer until the cauliflower is tender.

Nutritional Value:
- Calories: 320
- Protein: 12g
- Sodium: 150mg
- Phosphorus: 180mg
- Potassium: 500mg

Cooking Duration :30 minutes

3. Lemon Garlic Grilled Chicken

Ingredients:
- 4 boneless, skinless chicken breasts
- 2 tablespoons olive oil
- 2 cloves garlic, minced
- 1 lemon (juiced)
- 1 teaspoon dried oregano
- Salt and pepper to taste

Preparation:
1. Preheat the grill to medium-high heat.

2. Mix olive oil, garlic, lemon juice, oregano, salt, and pepper.

3. Brush the mixture over chicken breasts and grill for 6-8 minutes per side.

Nutritional Value:
- Calories: 280
- Protein: 35g
- Sodium: 90mg
- Phosphorus: 250mg
- Potassium: 400mg

Cooking Duration :16 minutes

4. Vegetarian Quinoa Stuffed Bell Peppers

Ingredients:
- 4 bell peppers, halved and seeds removed
- 1 cup of quinoa
- 2 cup of vegetable broth
- 1 can (15 oz) black beans, drained
- 1 cup of corn kernels
- 1 cup of tomatoes, diced
- 1 teaspoon cumin
- 1 teaspoon chili powder
- Salt and pepper to taste
- 1 cup of shredded low-fat cheese

Preparation:
1. Preheat the oven to 375°F (190°C).
2. Cook quinoa in vegetable broth according to package instructions.
3. In a bowl, combine quinoa, black beans, corn, tomatoes, cumin, chili powder, salt, and pepper.
4. Stuff bell peppers with the quinoa mixture, top with shredded cheese, and bake for 25-30 minutes.

Nutritional Value:
- Calories: 350
- Protein: 15g
- Sodium: 200mg
- Phosphorus: 180mg
- Potassium: 450mg

Cooking Duration :30 minutes

5. Salmon and Asparagus Foil Packets

Ingredients:
- 4 salmon fillets (6 oz each)
- 1 bunch asparagus, trimmed
- 2 tablespoons olive oil
- 2 cloves garlic, minced
- 1 lemon, sliced
- Salt and pepper to taste

Preparation:
1. Preheat the oven to 400°F (200°C).
2. Place each salmon fillet on a piece of foil.
3. Toss asparagus with olive oil, garlic, salt, and pepper, and place it next to the salmon.
4. Seal the foil packets and bake for 15-20 minutes.

Nutritional Value:
- Calories: 320
- Protein: 30g
- Sodium: 80mg
- Phosphorus: 250mg
- Potassium: 450mg

Cooking Duration :20 minutes

6. Mushroom and Spinach Risotto

Ingredients:
- 1 cup of Arborio rice
- 4 cup of low-sodium vegetable broth
- 1 onion, finely chopped
- 2 cloves garlic, minced
- 1 cup of mushrooms, sliced
- 2 cup of fresh spinach
- 1/2 cup of grated Parmesan cheese
- 2 tablespoons olive oil
- Salt and pepper to taste

Preparation:

1. In a pan, sauté the onion in olive oil until translucent.
2. Add garlic, mushrooms, and rice; cook until the rice is lightly browned.
3. Gradually add vegetable broth, stirring until absorbed.
4. Fold in spinach and Parmesan until creamy.

Nutritional Value:

- Calories: 280
- Protein: 10g
- Sodium: 200mg
- Phosphorus: 180mg
- Potassium: 350mg

Cooking Duration :35 minutes

7. Turkey and Vegetable Chili

Ingredients:

- 1 pound ground turkey
- 1 onion, diced
- 2 bell peppers, diced
- 2 cans (15 oz each) low-sodium kidney beans, drained
- 1 can (28 oz) crushed tomatoes
- 1 cup of corn kernels
- 2 tablespoons chili powder
- 1 teaspoon cumin

- Salt and pepper to taste

Preparation:
1. In a pot, brown the ground turkey with onions and bell peppers.
2. Add kidney beans, crushed tomatoes, corn, chili powder, cumin, salt, and pepper.
3. Simmer for 25-30 minutes.

Nutritional Value:
- Calories: 320
- Protein: 25g
- Sodium: 250mg
- Phosphorus: 200mg
- Potassium: 500mg

Cooking Duration :30 minutes

8. Eggplant Parmesan

Ingredients:
- 2 large eggplants, sliced
- 2 cup of low-sodium marinara sauce
- 2 cup of part-skim mozzarella cheese, shredded
- 1 cup of grated Parmesan cheese
- 1 cup of whole wheat breadcrumbs
- 2 tablespoons olive oil
-1 teaspoon dried oregano
- Salt and pepper to taste

Preparation:
1. Preheat the oven to 375°F (190°C).
2. Brush eggplant slices with olive oil, coat with breadcrumbs, and bake until golden.
3. In a baking dish, layer marinara sauce, baked eggplant, mozzarella, and Parmesan. Repeat.
4. Sprinkle with oregano and bake for 25-30 minutes.

Nutritional Value:
- Calories: 300
- Protein: 15g
- Sodium: 300mg
- Phosphorus: 250mg
- Potassium: 450mg

Cooking Duration :30 minutes

9. Chicken and Broccoli Stir-Fry

Ingredients:
- 1-pound boneless, skinless chicken breasts, sliced
- 4 cup of broccoli florets
- 1 red bell pepper, sliced
- 1/2 cup of low-sodium soy sauce
- 2 tablespoons honey
- 1 tablespoon cornstarch
- 2 tablespoons sesame oil
- 2 cloves garlic, minced

Preparation:

1. In a wok or large skillet, heat sesame oil and sauté garlic.
2. Add chicken and cook until browned, then add broccoli and bell pepper.
3. In a bowl, mix soy sauce, honey, and cornstarch. Pour over chicken and vegetables, stir-fry until the sauce thickens.

Nutritional Value:

- Calories: 350
- Protein: 30g
- Sodium: 300mg
- Phosphorus: 200mg
- Potassium: 450mg

Cooking Duration :20 minutes

10. Greek Quinoa Salad with Grilled Shrimp

Ingredients:
- 1 pound shrimp, peeled and deveined
- 1 cup of quinoa
- 2 cup of water
- 1 cucumber, diced
- 1 cup of cherry tomatoes, halved
- 1/2 cup of Kalamata olives, pitted and sliced
- 1/2 cup of crumbled feta cheese
- 2 tablespoons olive oil
- 1 lemon (juiced)
- 1 teaspoon dried oregano
- Salt and pepper to taste

Preparation:
1. Cook quinoa in water according to package instructions.
2. Season shrimp with olive oil, lemon juice, oregano, salt, and pepper. Grill until pink.
3. In a bowl, combine cooked quinoa, cucumber, tomatoes, olives, feta, and grilled shrimp.

Nutritional Value:
- Calories: 380
- Protein: 30g
- Sodium: 350mg
- Phosphorus: 250mg

- Potassium: 450mg

Cooking Duration :25 minutes

Please note that these recipes are general suggestions, and individuals with kidney disease should consult with their healthcare provider or a registered dietitian for personalized dietary advice. Adjustments may be necessary based on individual dietary restrictions and health conditions.

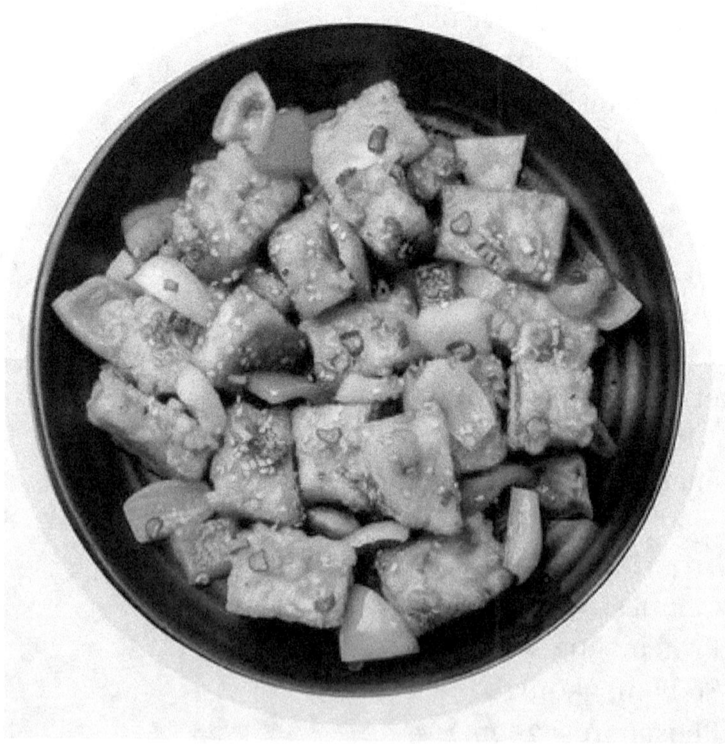

10 KIDNEY DISEASE DESSERT RECIPES

Ten kidney-friendly dessert recipes featuring detailed ingredients, preparation steps, measurements, nutritional details, and cooking durations.

1. Baked Apples with Cinnamon and Walnuts

Ingredients:
- 4 medium apples
- 1/4 cup of walnuts, chopped
- 2 tablespoons honey
- 1 teaspoon ground cinnamon

Preparation:
1. Preheat the oven to 375°F (190°C).
2. Core the apples and place them in a baking dish.
3. In a bowl, combine walnuts, honey, and cinnamon.
4. Fill each apple with the mixture.
5. Bake for 25-30 minutes or until the apples are tender.

Nutritional Value:
- Calories: 150
- Protein: 2g
- Sodium: 0mg
- Phosphorus: 40mg
- Potassium: 200mg

Cooking Duration :30 minutes

2. Mixed Berry Parfait

Ingredients:
- 2 cup of mixed berries (strawberries, blueberries, raspberries)
- 1 cup of low-fat Greek yogurt
- 2 tablespoons honey
- 1/4 cup of granola

Preparation:
1. Rinse and prepare the berries.
2. Layer berries, yogurt, honey, and granola in serving glasses.
3. Repeat the layers.
4. Chill in the refrigerator for at least 1 hour before serving.

Nutritional Value:
- Calories: 200
- Protein: 8g
- Sodium: 30mg
- Phosphorus: 150mg
- Potassium: 250mg

Cooking Duration :10 minutes

3. Peach and Almond Crisp

Ingredients:
- 4 cup of sliced peaches (fresh or canned in juice)
- 1/2 cup of almond flour
- 1/4 cup of rolled oats
- 2 tablespoons honey
- 1/2 teaspoon ground cinnamon

Preparation:
1. Preheat the oven to 375°F (190°C).
2. Place sliced peaches in a baking dish.
3. Mix almond flour, oats, honey, and cinnamon in a bowl.
4. Sprinkle the mixture over the peaches.
5. Bake for 25-30 minutes or until the topping is golden.

Nutritional Value:
- Calories: 180
- Protein: 4g
- Sodium: 0mg
- Phosphorus: 70mg
- Potassium: 220mg

Cooking Duration :30 minutes

4. Vanilla Chia Pudding with Fresh Berries

Ingredients:
- 1/4 cup of chia seeds
- 1 cup of unsweetened almond milk
- 1 teaspoon vanilla extract
- 1 tablespoon maple syrup
- 1 cup of fresh berries (strawberries, blueberries)

Preparation:
1. Mix chia seeds, almond milk, vanilla extract, and maple syrup in a bowl.
2. Refrigerate for at least 2 hours or overnight.
3. Stir well before serving and top with fresh berries.

Nutritional Value:
- Calories: 150
- Protein: 4g
- Sodium: 70mg
- Phosphorus: 80mg
- Potassium: 120mg

Cooking Duration :2 hours (including chilling time)

5. Banana-Oat Cookies

Ingredients:
- 2 ripe bananas, mashed
- 1 cup of rolled oats
- 1/4 cup of chopped nuts (walnuts or almonds)
- 1/4 cup of raisins
- 1/2 teaspoon vanilla extract

Preparation:
1. Preheat the oven to 350°F (175°C).
2. Combine mashed bananas, oats, nuts, raisins, and vanilla extract in a bowl.
3. Drop spoonful of the mixture onto a baking sheet.
4. Bake for 15-20 minutes or until the edges are golden.

Nutritional Value:
- Calories: 120
- Protein: 3g
- Sodium: 0mg
- Phosphorus: 80mg
- Potassium: 180mg

Cooking Duration :20 minutes

6. Coconut Rice Pudding

Ingredients:
- 1/2 cup of Arborio rice
- 2 cup of coconut milk (unsweetened)
- 1/4 cup of honey
- 1/4 cup of shredded coconut
- 1/2 teaspoon vanilla extract

Preparation:
1. Combine rice, coconut milk, honey, and shredded coconut in a saucepan.
2. Bring to a simmer over medium heat, then reduce heat to low.
3. Cook for 25-30 minutes, stirring occasionally, until rice is tender.
4. Remove from heat, stir in vanilla extract, and let it cool.

Nutritional Value:
- Calories: 220
- Protein: 3g
- Sodium: 10mg
- Phosphorus: 80mg
- Potassium: 100mg

Cooking Duration : 30 minutes

7. Frozen Banana Bites

Ingredients:
- 2 ripe bananas, sliced
- 1/4 cup of peanut butter
- 1/4 cup of dark chocolate chips
- 2 tablespoons chopped almonds

Preparation:
1. Line a tray with parchment paper.
2. Spread a thin layer of peanut butter on banana slices.
3. Create sandwiches with two slices and freeze for 1 hour.
4. Melt chocolate chips and dip each banana sandwich into the melted chocolate.
5. Sprinkle with chopped almonds and freeze for an additional 2 hours.

Nutritional Value:
- Calories: 180
- Protein: 3g
- Sodium: 20mg
- Phosphorus: 70mg
- Potassium: 300mg

Cooking Duration :3 hours (including freezing time

8. Cinnamon Baked Pears

Ingredients:
- 4 ripe pears, halved and cored
- 1 tablespoon honey
- 1/2 teaspoon ground cinnamon
- 1/4 cup of chopped pecans

Preparation:
1. Preheat the oven to 375°F (190°C).
2. Place pear halves in a baking dish.
3. Drizzle honey over the pears and sprinkle with cinnamon.
4. Bake for 20-25 minutes or until pears are tender.
5. Garnish with chopped pecans before serving.

Nutritional Value:
- Calories: 150
- Protein: 1g
- Sodium: 0mg
- Phosphorus: 30mg
- Potassium: 200mg

Cooking Duration :25 minutes

9. Avocado Chocolate Mousse

Ingredients:
- 2 ripe avocados
- 1/4 cup of unsweetened cocoa powder
- 1/4 cup of honey
- 1 teaspoon vanilla extract
- 1/4 cup of almond milk

Preparation:
1. In a blender, combine avocados, cocoa powder, honey, vanilla extract, and almond milk.
2. Blend until smooth and creamy.
3. Chill in the refrigerator for at least 1 hour before serving.

Nutritional Value:
- Calories: 200
- Protein: 3g
- Sodium: 10mg
- Phosphorus: 70mg
- Potassium: 450mg

Cooking Duration :10 minutes

10. Chia Seed and Berry Jam

Ingredients:
- 2 cup of mixed berries (strawberries, blueberries, raspberries)
- 2 tablespoons chia seeds
- 2 tablespoons honey
- 1/2 teaspoon vanilla extract

Preparation:
1. In a saucepan, heat berries over medium heat until they begin to break down.
2. Mash the berries with a fork or potato masher.
3. Stir in chia seeds, honey, and vanilla extract.
4. Simmer for an additional 10 minutes until the jam thickens.
5. Let it cool before transferring to a jar and refrigerating.

Nutritional Value:
- Calories: 80
- Protein: 1g
- Sodium: 0mg
- Phosphorus: 20mg
- Potassium: 100mg

Cooking Duration :20 minutes

10 KIDNEY DISEASE SNACKS RECIPES.

Ten snack recipes suitable for those with kidney conditions. Each recipe includes a list of ingredients, detailed preparation methods, quantities, nutritional information, and cooking times.

1. Hummus and Veggie Sticks

Ingredients:
- 1 can (15 oz) low-sodium chickpeas, drained
- 2 tablespoons tahini
- 2 cloves garlic, minced
- 2 tablespoons olive oil
- Juice of 1 lemon
- Carrot and cucumber stick for dipping

Preparation:
1. In a blender, combine chickpeas, tahini, garlic, olive oil, and lemon juice.
2. Blend until smooth.
3. Serve with carrot and cucumber sticks.

Nutritional Information:
- Calories: 150
- Protein: 5g
- Sodium: 50mg
- Phosphorus: 80mg
- Potassium: 180mg

Cooking Duration :10 minutes

2. Greek Yogurt Parfait

Ingredients:
- 1 cup of low-fat Greek yogurt
- 1/4 cup of granola
- 1/2 cup of mixed berries (strawberries, blueberries)
- 1 tablespoon honey

Preparation:
1. In a glass, layer Greek yogurt, granola, and mixed berries.
2. Repeat the layers.
3. Drizzle with honey before serving.

Nutritional Information:
- Calories: 200
- Protein: 15g
- Sodium: 50mg
- Phosphorus: 150mg
- Potassium: 250mg

Cooking Duration :5 minutes

3. Cucumber and Cream Cheese Roll-Ups

Ingredients:
- 1 large cucumber, thinly sliced lengthwise
- 4 ounces low-fat cream cheese
- 1 tablespoon fresh dill, chopped
- Smoked salmon slices (optional)

Preparation:
1. In a bowl, mix cream cheese and dill.
2. Spread the mixture on cucumber slices.
3. Add smoked salmon if desired and roll up.

Nutritional Information:
- Calories: 120
- Protein: 6g
- Sodium: 80mg
- Phosphorus: 100mg
- Potassium: 250mg

Cooking Duration :10 minutes

4. Roasted Chickpeas

Ingredients:
- 1 can (15 oz) chickpeas, drained and rinsed
- 1 tablespoon olive oil
- 1 teaspoon ground cumin
- 1/2 teaspoon smoked paprika
- Salt to taste

Preparation:
1. Preheat the oven to 400°F (200°C).
2. Pat chickpeas dry and toss with olive oil, cumin, paprika, and salt.
3. Spread on a baking sheet and roast for 20-25 minutes.

Nutritional Information:
- Calories: 150
- Protein: 6g
- Sodium: 150mg
- Phosphorus: 100mg
- Potassium: 180mg

Cooking Duration :25 minutes

5. Cheese and Whole Grain Crackers

Ingredients:
- 1-ounce low-fat cheese (cheddar, mozzarella)
- 10 whole-grain crackers

Preparation:
1. Slice cheese into cubes.
2. Serve with whole-grain crackers.

Nutritional Information:
- Calories: 200
- Protein: 10g
- Sodium: 150mg
- Phosphorus: 100mg
- Potassium: 50mg

Cooking Duration :5 minutes

6. Fruit Kabobs with Mint Yogurt Dip

Ingredients:
- 1 cup of mixed fruit (melon, berries, grapes)
- 1 cup of low-fat vanilla yogurt
- Fresh mint leaves

Preparation:
1. Thread mixed fruit onto skewers.

2. In a bowl, mix yogurt and chopped mint.
3. Serve fruit kabobs with mint yogurt dip.

Nutritional Information:
- Calories: 150
- Protein: 5g
- Sodium: 80mg
- Phosphorus: 120mg
- Potassium: 200mg

Cooking Duration :10 minutes

7. Apple and Almond Butter Sandwiches

Ingredients:
- 1 medium apple, sliced
- 2 tablespoons almond butter
- 1 tablespoon raisins

Preparation:
1. Spread almond butter on apple slices.
2. Sandwich them together and press raisins on top.

Nutritional Information:
- Calories: 200
- Protein: 4g
- Sodium: 0mg
- Phosphorus: 80mg

- Potassium: 200mg

Cooking Duration :5 minutes

8. Vegetable Salsa with Baked Pita Chips

Ingredients:
- 2 tomatoes, diced
- 1/2 red onion, finely chopped
- 1 bell pepper, diced
- 1/4 cup of fresh cilantro, chopped
- 1 lime (juiced)
- Whole wheat pita, cut into triangles

Preparation:
1. In a bowl, combine tomatoes, red onion, bell pepper, cilantro, and lime juice.
2. Arrange pita triangles on a baking sheet and bake at 350°F (175°C) for 10 minutes.
3. Serve pita chips with vegetable salsa.

Nutritional Information:
- Calories: 180
- Protein: 5g
- Sodium: 200mg
- Phosphorus: 100mg
- Potassium: 300mg

Cooking Duration :15 minutes

9. Edamame Guacamole

Ingredients:
- 1 cup of edamame, shelled
- 1 avocado, mashed
- 1 clove garlic, minced
- 1 tablespoon lime juice
- Salt and pepper to taste

Preparation:
1. Cook edamame in boiling water for 5 minutes, then drain.
2. In a blender, combine edamame, mashed avocado, garlic, lime juice, salt, and pepper.
3. Blend until smooth.

Nutritional Information:
- Calories: 180
- Protein: 9g
- Sodium: 10mg
- Phosphorus: 120mg
- Potassium: 450mg

Cooking Duration :15 minutes

10. Trail Mix with Dried Fruits and Nuts

Ingredients:
- 1/2 cup of almonds
- 1/2 cup of walnuts
- 1/4 cup of pumpkin seeds
- 1/4 cup of dried apricots, chopped
- 1/4 cup of dried cranberries
- 1/4 cup of dark chocolate chips

Preparation:
1. Mix almonds, walnuts, pumpkin seeds, dried apricots, dried cranberries, and dark chocolate chips in a bowl.
2. Store in an airtight container for a ready-to-eat snack.

Nutritional Information:
- Calories: 250
- Protein: 8g
- Sodium: 5mg
- Phosphorus: 150mg
- Potassium: 300mg

Cooking Duration :5 minutes

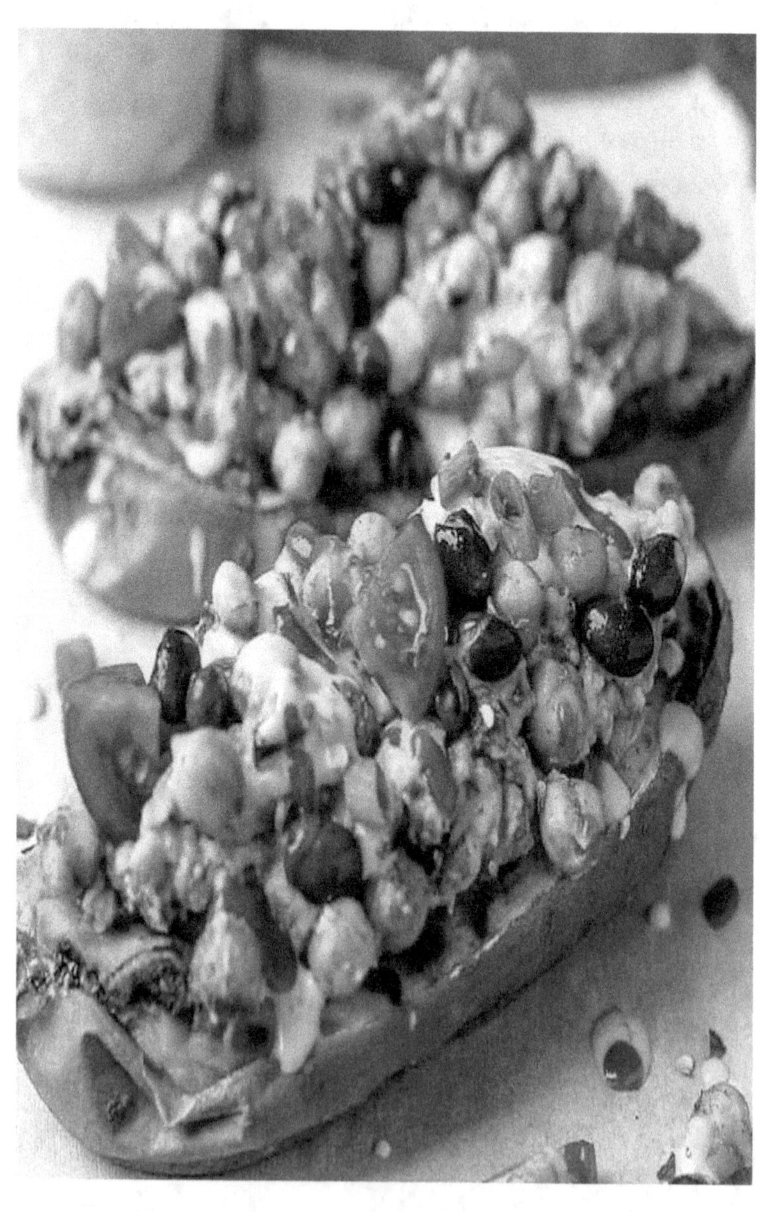

10 KIDNEY DISEASE SMOOTHIE RECIPES.

Ten kidney-friendly smoothie recipes with detailed ingredients, preparation methods, quantities, nutritional information, and cooking times:

1. Berry Blast Smoothie

Ingredients:
- 1/2 cup of fresh blueberries
- 1/2 cup of hulled strawberries
- 1/4 cup of raspberries
- 1/2 banana
- 1 cup of low-fat yogurt
- 1 tablespoon honey
- 1/2 cup of ice cubes

Preparation:
1. Place blueberries, strawberries, raspberries, banana, yogurt, honey, and ice cubes in a blender.
2. Blend until smooth.
3. Pour into a glass and serve.

Nutritional Value:
- Calories: 180
- Protein: 8g
- Sodium: 50mg
- Phosphorus: 150mg
- Potassium: 250mg

Cooking Duration :5 minutes

2. Green Goodness Smoothie

Ingredients:
- 1 cup of fresh spinach leaves
- 1/2 cucumber, peeled and sliced
- 1/2 green apple, cored and chopped
- Juice of 1/2 lemon
- 1/2 cup of water
- 1 tablespoon chia seeds
- 1/2 cup of ice cubes

Preparation:
1. Combine spinach, cucumber, apple, lemon juice, water, chia seeds, and ice cubes in a blender.
2. Blend until smooth.
3. Pour into a glass and enjoy.

Nutritional Value:
- Calories: 120
- Protein: 5g
- Sodium: 30mg
- Phosphorus: 120mg
- Potassium: 300mg

Cooking Duration :5 minutes

3. Tropical Delight Smoothie

Ingredients:
- 1/2 cup of pineapple chunks
- 1/2 cup of mango chunks
- 1/2 banana
- 1/2 cup of coconut water
- 1/4 cup of Greek yogurt
- 1 tablespoon flaxseeds
- 1/2 cup of ice cubes

Preparation:
1. Combine pineapple, mango, banana, coconut water, Greek yogurt, flaxseeds, and ice cubes in a blender.
2. Blend until smooth.
3. Pour into a glass and serve.

Nutritional Value:
- Calories: 200
- Protein: 7g
- Sodium: 20mg
- Phosphorus: 100mg
- Potassium: 350mg

Cooking Duration :5 minutes

4. Creamy Avocado Spinach Smoothie

Ingredients:
- 1/2 avocado
- 1 cup of fresh spinach leaves
- 1/2 cup of cucumber, sliced
- Juice of 1/2 lime
- 1/2 cup of unsweetened almond milk
- 1 tablespoon hemp seeds
- 1/2 cup of ice cubes

Preparation:
1. In a blender, combine avocado, spinach, cucumber, lime juice, almond milk, hemp seeds, and ice cubes.
2. Blend until smooth.
3. Pour into a glass and enjoy.

Nutritional Value:
- Calories: 220
- Protein: 6g
- Sodium: 60mg
- Phosphorus: 140mg
- Potassium: 450mg

Cooking Duration :5 minutes

5. Banana Berry Protein Smoothie

Ingredients:
- 1/2 banana
- 1/2 cup of mixed berries (strawberries, blueberries)
- 1/2 cup of low-fat yogurt
- 1/2 cup of milk (skim or almond)
- 1 scoop protein powder
- 1 tablespoon almond butter
- 1/2 cup of ice cubes

Preparation:
1. Combine banana, mixed berries, yogurt, milk, protein powder, almond butter, and ice cubes in a blender.
2. Blend until smooth.
3. Pour into a glass and serve.

Nutritional Value:
- Calories: 250
- Protein: 15g
- Sodium: 70mg
- Phosphorus: 200mg
- Potassium: 350mg

Cooking Duration :5 minutes

6. Peachy Oat Smoothie

Ingredients:
- 1/2 cup of sliced peaches (fresh or canned in juice)
- 1/4 cup of rolled oats
- 1/2 cup of low-fat Greek yogurt
- 1 tablespoon honey
- 1/2 teaspoon vanilla extract
- 1/2 cup of ice cubes

Preparation:
1. In a blender, combine peaches, rolled oats, Greek yogurt, honey, vanilla extract, and ice cubes.
2. Blend until smooth.
3. Pour into a glass and enjoy.

Nutritional Value:
- Calories: 180
- Protein: 8g
- Sodium: 40mg
- Phosphorus: 130mg
- Potassium: 250mg

Cooking Duration :5 minutes

7. Strawberry Kiwi Citrus Smoothie

Ingredients:
- 1/2 cup of strawberries, hulled
- 1 kiwi, peeled and sliced
- Juice of 1/2 orange
- 1/2 cup of coconut water
- 1/4 cup of plain yogurt
- 1 tablespoon chia seeds
- 1/2 cup of ice cubes

Preparation:
1. Combine strawberries, kiwi, orange juice, coconut water, yogurt, chia seeds, and ice cubes in a blender.
2. Blend until smooth.
3. Pour into a glass and serve.

Nutritional Value:
- Calories: 150
- Protein: 5g
- Sodium: 30mg
- Phosphorus: 100mg
- Potassium: 300mg

Cooking Duration :5 minutes

8. Cherry Almond Spinach Smoothie

Ingredients:
- 1/2 cup of cherries, pitted
- 1/4 cup of almonds
- 1 cup of fresh spinach leaves
- 1/2 cup of unsweetened almond milk
- 1 tablespoon flaxseeds
- 1/2 cup of ice cubes

Preparation:
1. In a blender, combine cherries, almonds, spinach, almond milk, flaxseeds, and ice cubes.
2. Blend until smooth.
3. Pour into a glass and enjoy.

Nutritional Value:
- Calories: 200
- Protein: 7g
- Sodium: 40mg
- Phosphorus: 120mg
- Potassium: 300mg

Cooking Duration :5 minutes

9. Mango Coconut Protein Smoothie

Ingredients:
- 1/2 cup of mango chunks
- 1/4 cup of shredded coconut
- 1/2 cup of low-fat Greek yogurt
- 1/2 cup of unsweetened coconut milk
- 1 scoop protein powder
- 1 tablespoon chia seeds
- 1/2 cup of ice cubes

Preparation:
1. Combine mango chunks, shredded coconut, Greek yogurt, coconut milk, protein powder, chia seeds, and ice cubes in a blender.
2. Blend until smooth.
3. Pour into a glass and serve.

Nutritional Value:
- Calories: 220
- Protein: 15g
- Sodium: 50mg
- Phosphorus: 180mg
- Potassium: 350mg

Cooking Duration :5 minutes

10. Vanilla Almond Banana Smoothie

Ingredients:
- 1/2 banana
- 1/4 cup of almonds
- 1 cup of low-fat milk
- 1/2 teaspoon vanilla extract
- 1 tablespoon honey
- 1/2 cup of ice cubes

Preparation:
1. Combine banana, almonds, milk, vanilla extract, honey, and ice cubes in a blender.
2. Blend until smooth.
3. Pour into a glass and enjoy.

Nutritional Value:
- Calories: 200
- Protein: 9g
- Sodium: 60mg
- Phosphorus: 160mg
- Potassium: 300mg

Cooking Duration :5 minutes

CONCLUSION

In conclusion, this cookbook dedicated to kidney health stands as a valuable repository, presenting individuals with kidney conditions a diverse and delectable assortment of recipes meticulously crafted to align with their specific dietary requirements. The careful consideration given to ingredients, portion sizes, and nutritional details underscores a steadfast commitment to bolstering kidney health through a repertoire of flavorful and nourishing meals.

From nutrient-rich salads to gratifying main courses and enticing desserts, this cookbook not only addresses the nutritional needs of those with kidney disease but also transforms the pursuit of a kidney-friendly diet into a pleasurable and appealing venture. Through the strategic emphasis on low-sodium, low-phosphorus, and kidney-conscious ingredients, these recipes are thoughtfully constructed to contribute positively to overall kidney function.

The incorporation of comprehensive nutritional information empowers individuals to make educated choices, advocating for a proactive approach to their health management. The seamless alignment with established dietary guidelines for kidney disease, including prudent portion control, mindful sodium intake, and hydration considerations, reinforces the cookbook's dedication to supporting kidney wellness.

More than just a collection of recipes, this cookbook urges readers to perceive it as a companion in their wellness journey—a manual for adopting a lifestyle that nurtures kidney health. By embracing and adjusting to the principles elucidated in this cookbook, individuals aren't merely altering their immediate dietary habits; they are laying the groundwork for enduring well-being.

As you venture into this gastronomic odyssey, recognize that each dish marks a stride toward enhanced kidney health. Embrace the positive transformations in your diet as an investment in your long-term well-being. To echo the wisdom of Hippocrates, "Let food be thy medicine, and medicine be thy food." Your expedition to kidney health commences with each delectable and nutritious choice.

We extend our gratitude for selecting this cookbook as a guide on your journey to wellness. Relish every moment in the kitchen and savor the delightful flavors on your plate. Your feedback is immensely valued, so please take a moment to review and share your thoughts. Happy cooking, and here's to your kidney health!

THANK YOU!!!

IF YOU FIND THIS BOOK TO BE INFORMATIVE, INSPIRING, OR SIMPLY ENJOYABLE, I WOULD BE IMMENSELY GRATEFUL IF YOU COULD SHARE YOUR THOUGHTS WITH OTHERS. YOUR HONEST REVIEW CAN MAKE A DIFFERENCE IN HELPING MORE INDIVIDUALS DISCOVER THE BENEFITS OF A NOURISHING AND MINDFUL APPROACH TO EATING. PLEASE CONSIDER LEAVING A REVIEW ON AMAZON AND SHARE YOUR EXPERIENCE.

THANK YOU ONCE AGAIN FOR CHOOSING THIS BOOK AS A COMPANION ON YOUR PATH TO A HEALTHIER, HAPPIER YOU.

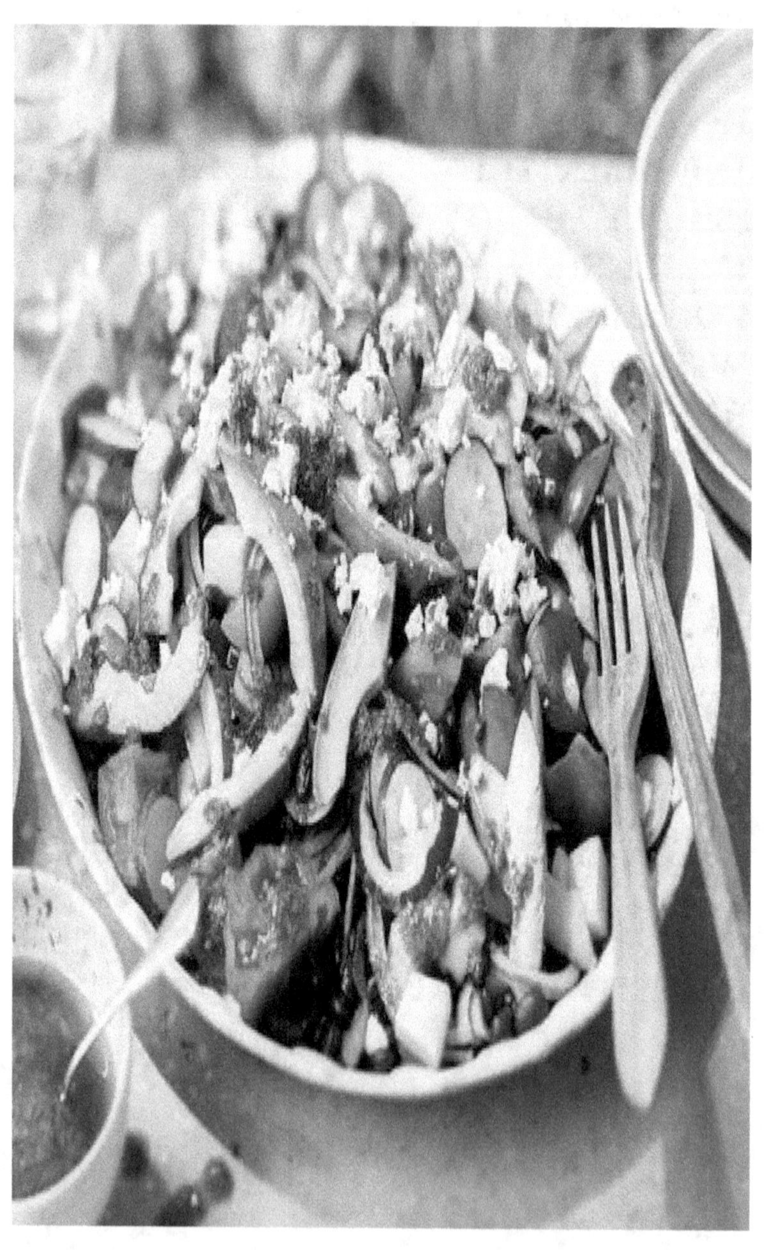

28 WEEKS RENAL DIET MEAL PLANNER

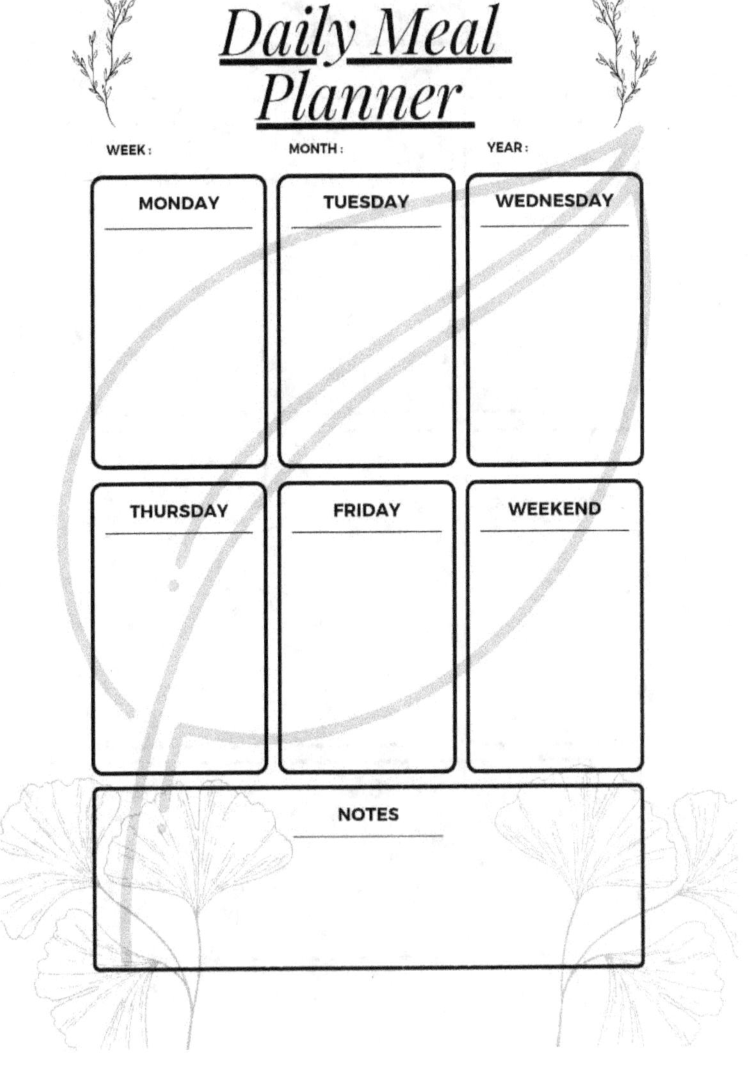

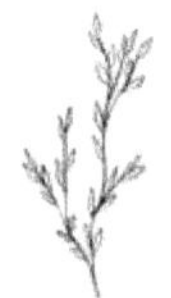
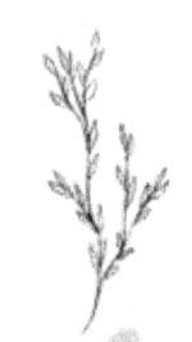

Daily Meal
Planner

WEEK: **MONTH:**   **YEAR:**

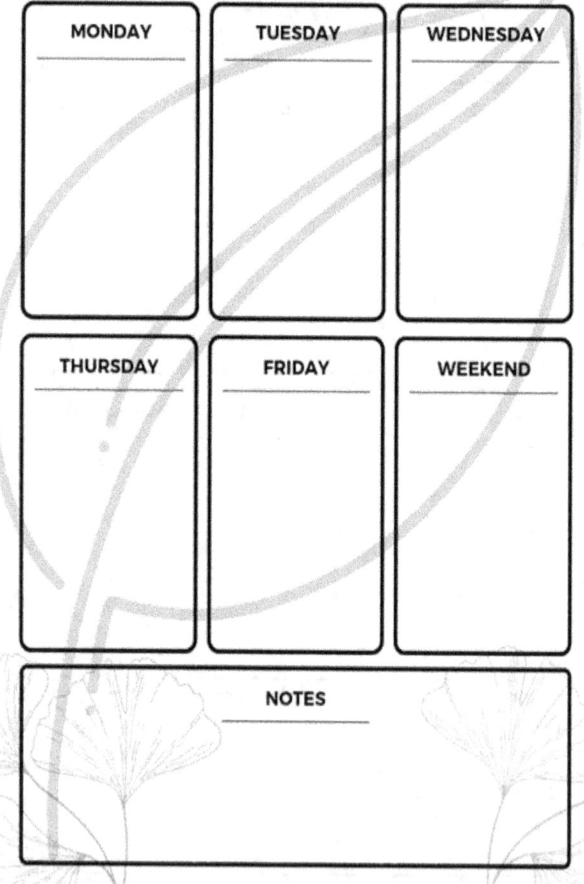

MONDAY	**TUESDAY**	**WEDNESDAY**

THURSDAY	**FRIDAY**	**WEEKEND**

NOTES

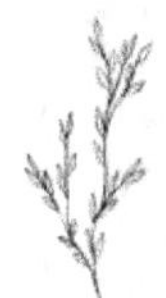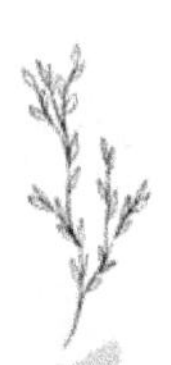

Daily Meal Planner

WEEK :   MONTH :   YEAR :

MONDAY	TUESDAY	WEDNESDAY

THURSDAY	FRIDAY	WEEKEND

NOTES

Daily Meal Planner

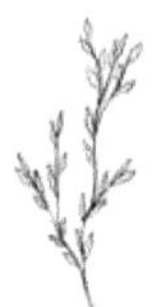

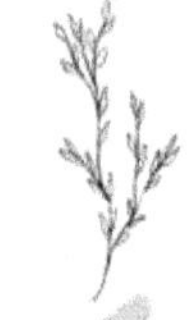

WEEK :   MONTH :   YEAR :

MONDAY	TUESDAY	WEDNESDAY

THURSDAY	FRIDAY	WEEKEND

NOTES

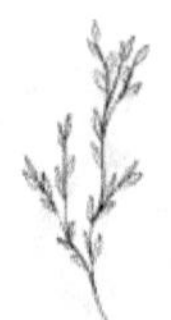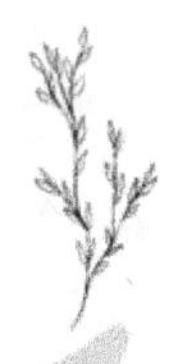

Daily Meal Planner

WEEK :   **MONTH :**   **YEAR :**

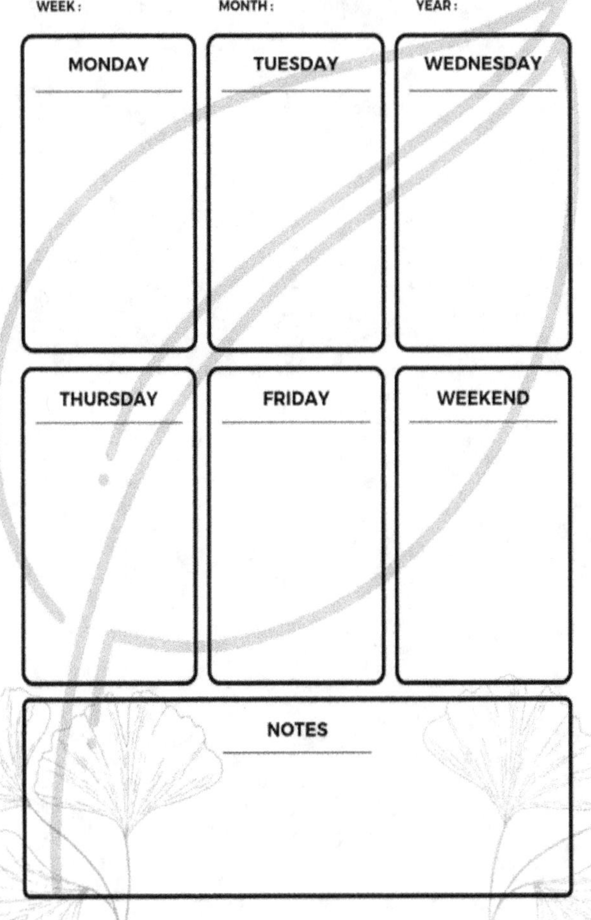

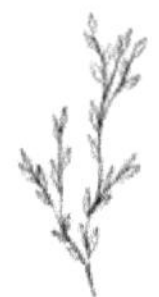
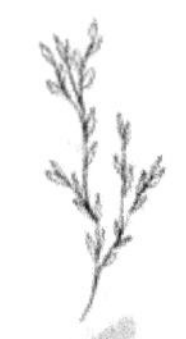

Daily Meal Planner

WEEK: **MONTH:**   **YEAR:**

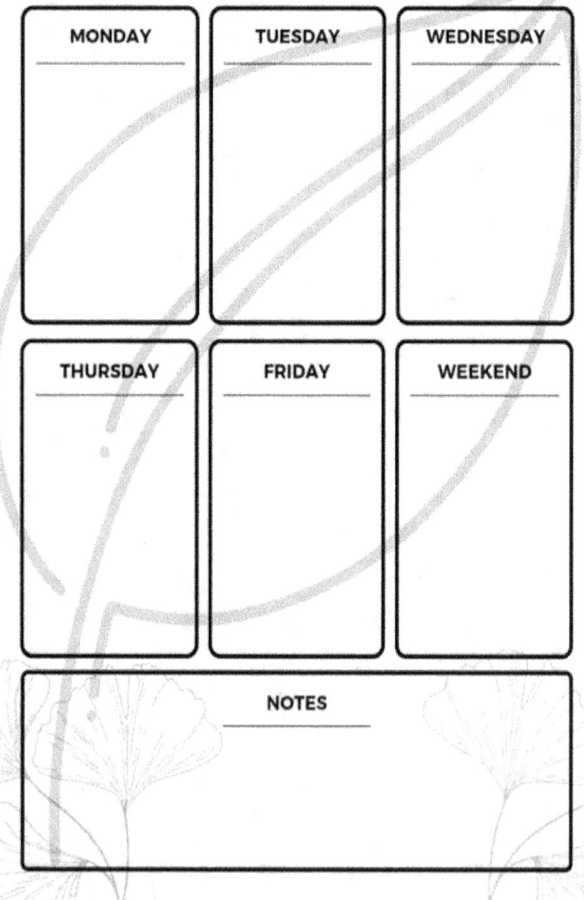

MONDAY	TUESDAY	WEDNESDAY

THURSDAY	FRIDAY	WEEKEND

NOTES

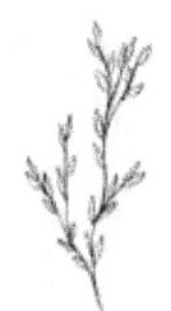 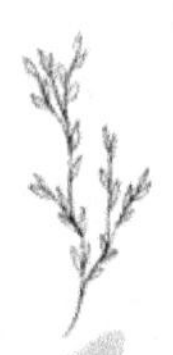

Daily Meal Planner

WEEK: **MONTH:**   **YEAR:**

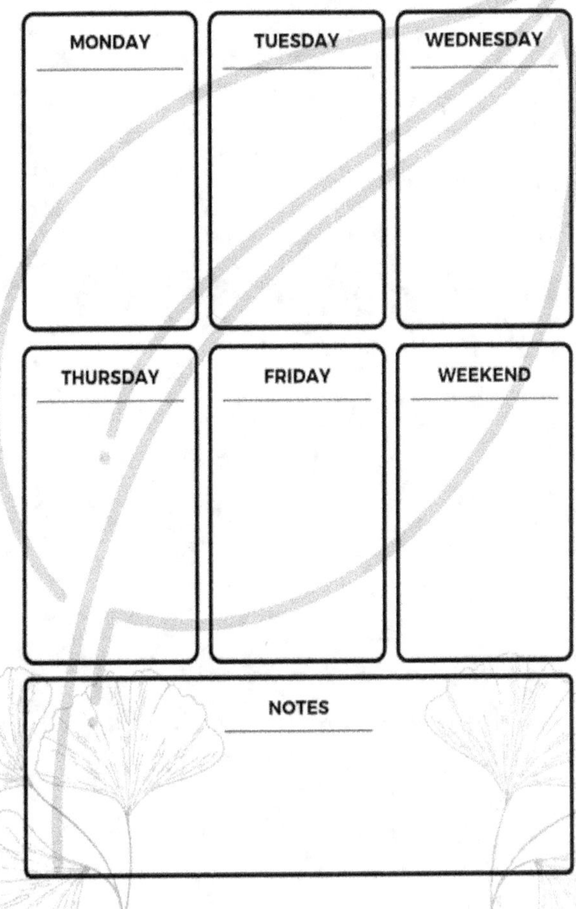

MONDAY	TUESDAY	WEDNESDAY

THURSDAY	FRIDAY	WEEKEND

NOTES

Daily Meal Planner

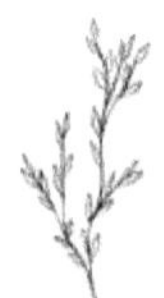 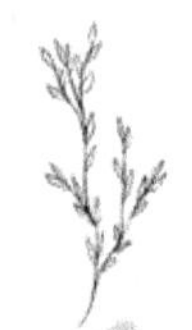

WEEK :   **MONTH :**   **YEAR :**

MONDAY	TUESDAY	WEDNESDAY

THURSDAY	FRIDAY	WEEKEND

NOTES

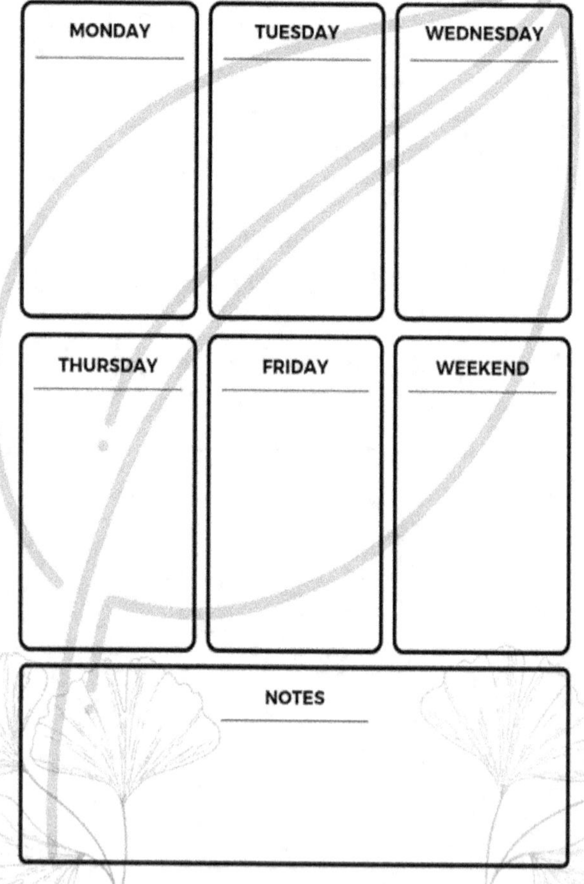

Daily Meal Planner

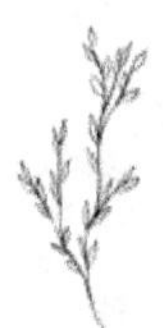
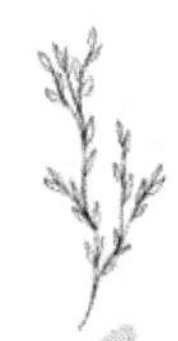

WEEK: **MONTH:**   **YEAR:**

MONDAY	TUESDAY	WEDNESDAY

THURSDAY	FRIDAY	WEEKEND

NOTES

Daily Meal Planner

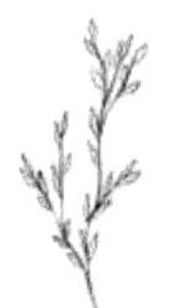
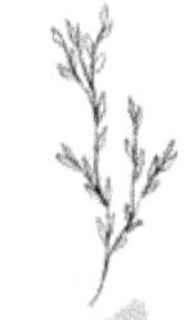

MONDAY	TUESDAY	WEDNESDAY

THURSDAY	FRIDAY	WEEKEND

NOTES

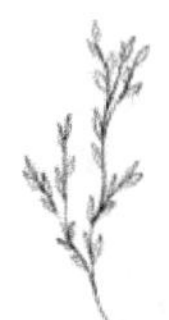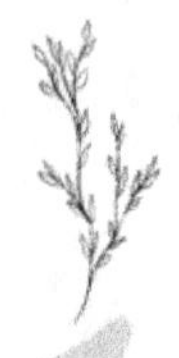

Daily Meal Planner

WEEK: **MONTH:**   **YEAR:**

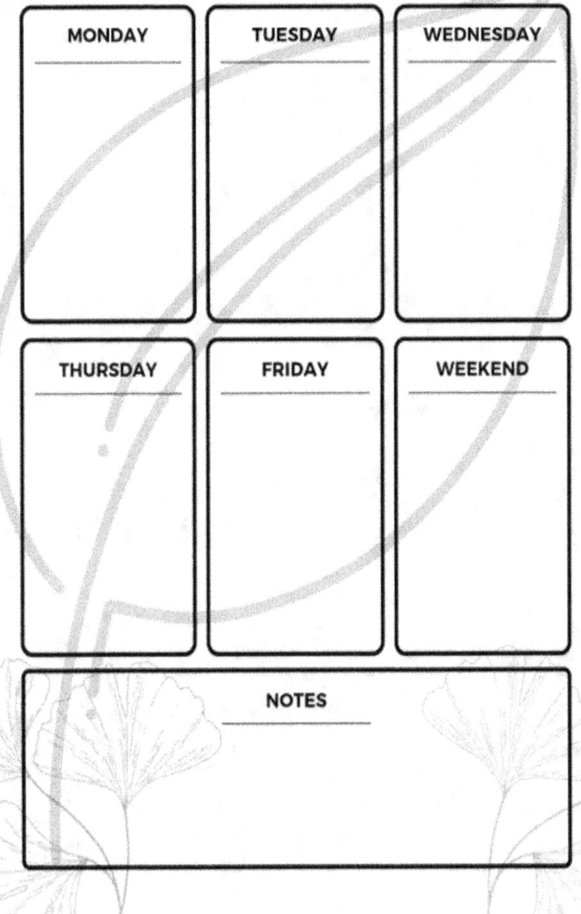

MONDAY	TUESDAY	WEDNESDAY

THURSDAY	FRIDAY	WEEKEND

NOTES

Daily Meal Planner

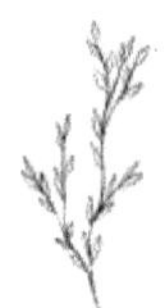
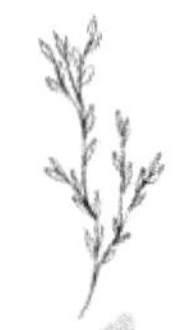

MONDAY	TUESDAY	WEDNESDAY

THURSDAY	FRIDAY	WEEKEND

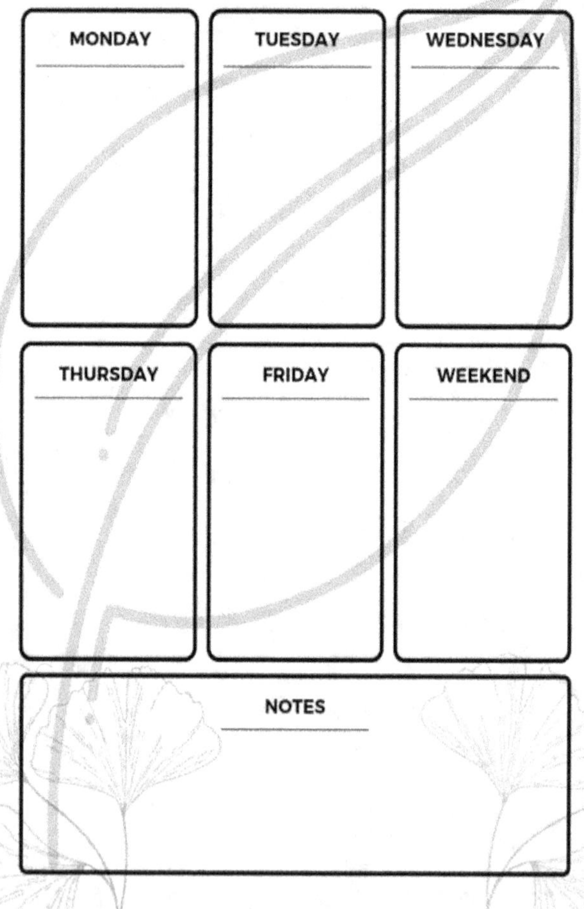

NOTES

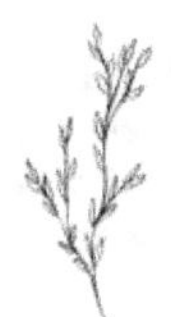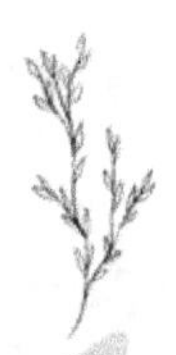

Daily Meal Planner

WEEK: **MONTH:**   **YEAR:**

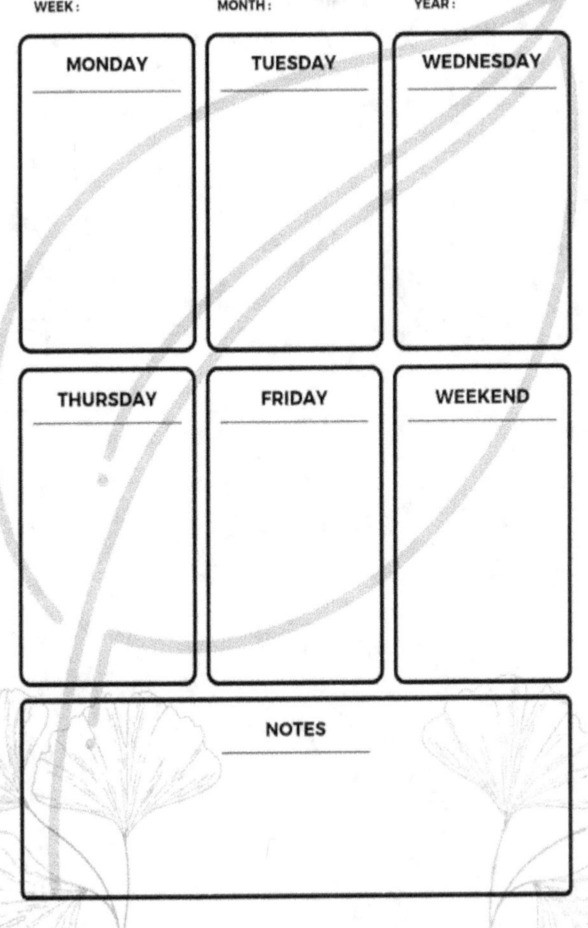

MONDAY	TUESDAY	WEDNESDAY

THURSDAY	FRIDAY	WEEKEND

NOTES

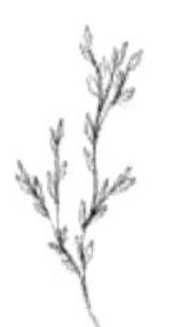

Daily Meal Planner

WEEK: **MONTH:** **YEAR:**

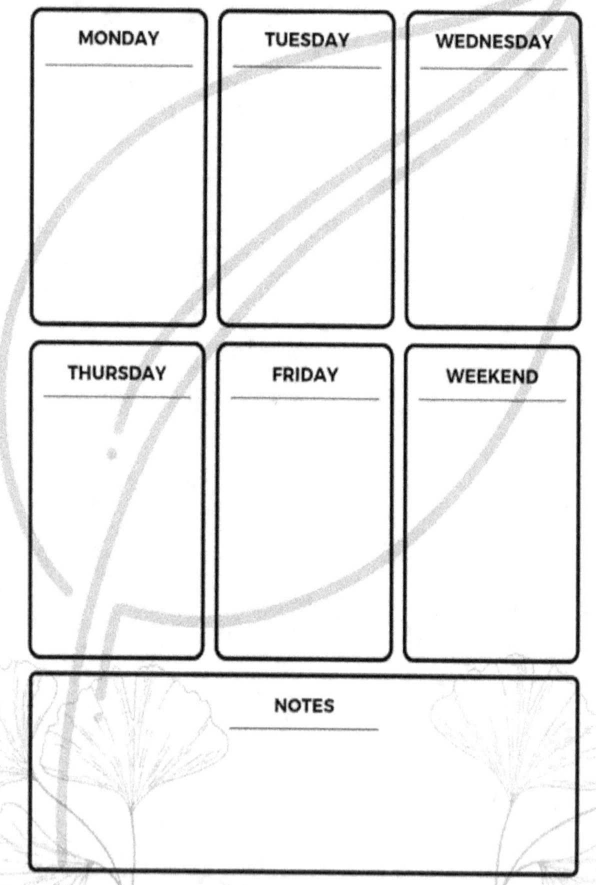

MONDAY	TUESDAY	WEDNESDAY

THURSDAY	FRIDAY	WEEKEND

NOTES

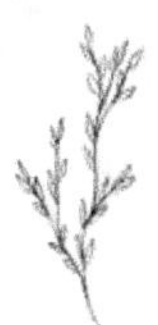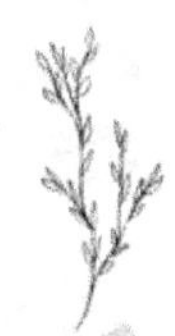

Daily Meal Planner

WEEK: MONTH: YEAR:

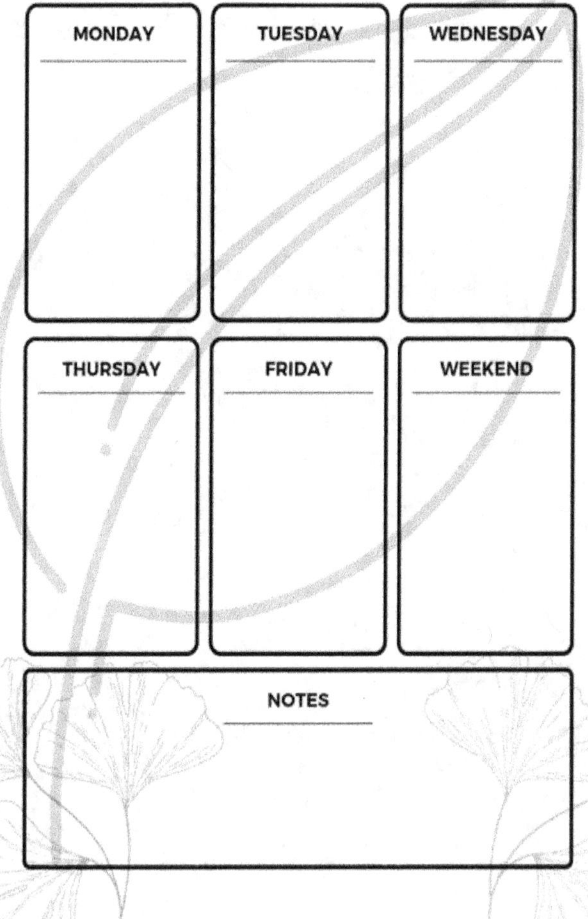

MONDAY	TUESDAY	WEDNESDAY

THURSDAY	FRIDAY	WEEKEND

NOTES

Daily Meal Planner

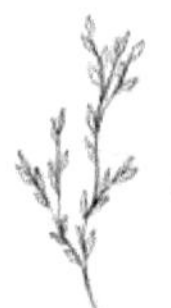 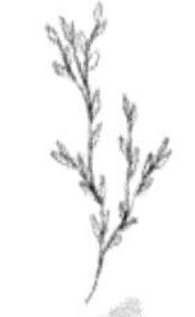

WEEK: MONTH: YEAR:

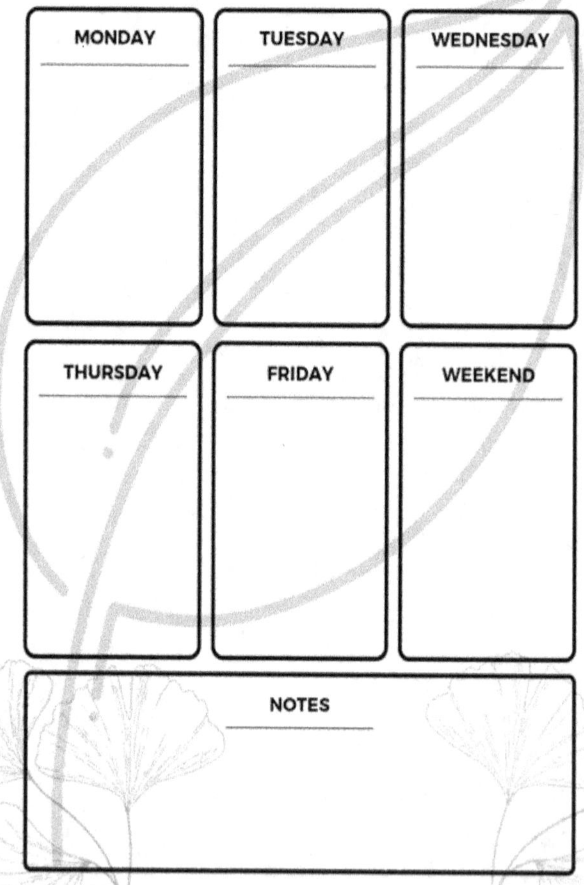

MONDAY	TUESDAY	WEDNESDAY

THURSDAY	FRIDAY	WEEKEND

NOTES

Daily Meal Planner

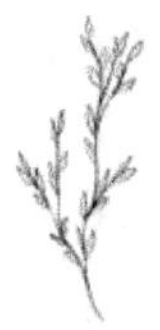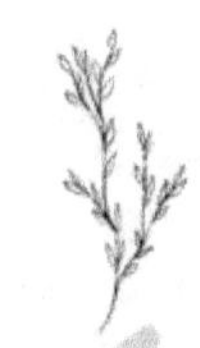

WEEK :   MONTH :   YEAR :

MONDAY	TUESDAY	WEDNESDAY

THURSDAY	FRIDAY	WEEKEND

NOTES

Daily Meal Planner

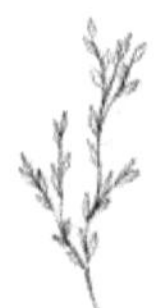
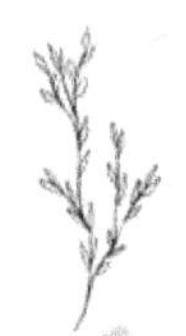

WEEK: MONTH: YEAR:

MONDAY	TUESDAY	WEDNESDAY

THURSDAY	FRIDAY	WEEKEND

NOTES

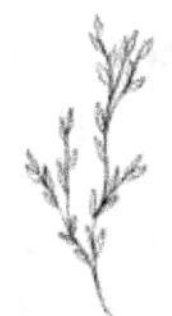
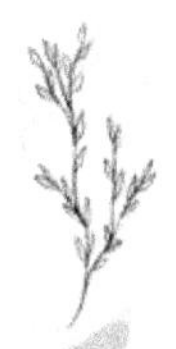

Daily Meal Planner

WEEK: **MONTH:**   **YEAR:**

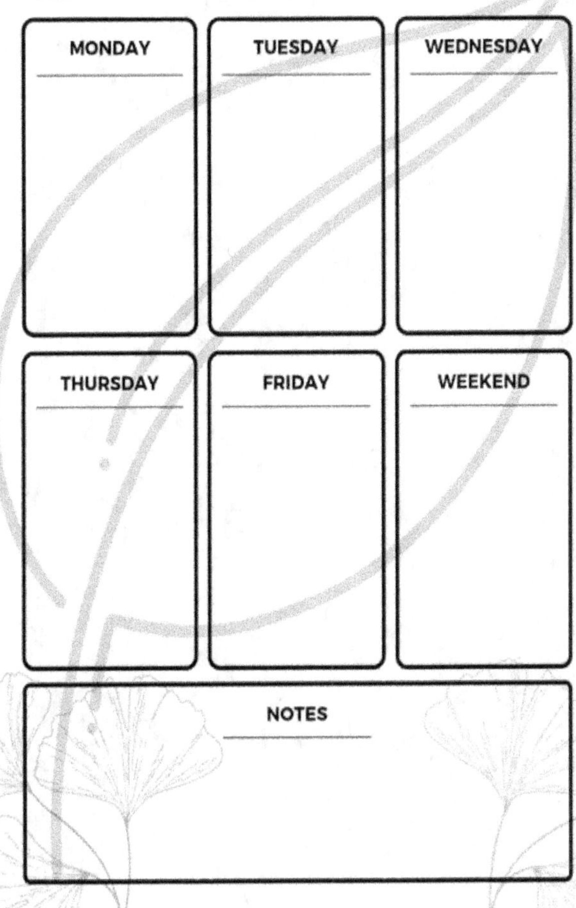

MONDAY

TUESDAY

WEDNESDAY

THURSDAY

FRIDAY

WEEKEND

NOTES

Daily Meal Planner

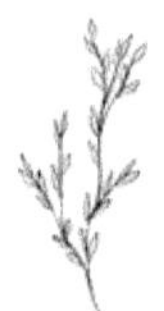

WEEK :   MONTH :   YEAR :

MONDAY	TUESDAY	WEDNESDAY

THURSDAY	FRIDAY	WEEKEND

NOTES

Daily Meal Planner

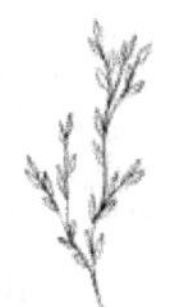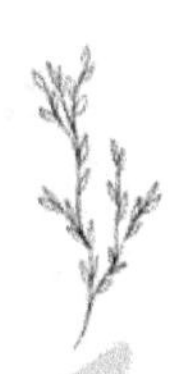

WEEK: MONTH: YEAR:

MONDAY	TUESDAY	WEDNESDAY

THURSDAY	FRIDAY	WEEKEND

NOTES

Daily Meal Planner

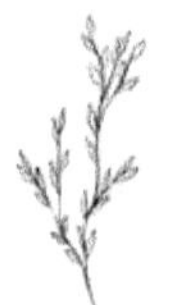

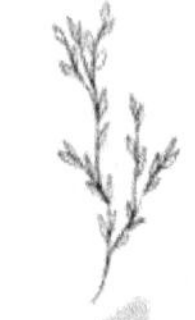

WEEK: MONTH: YEAR:

MONDAY

TUESDAY

WEDNESDAY

THURSDAY

FRIDAY

WEEKEND

NOTES

Daily Meal Planner

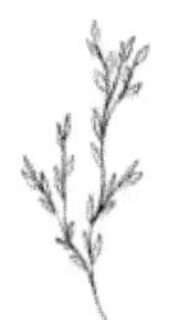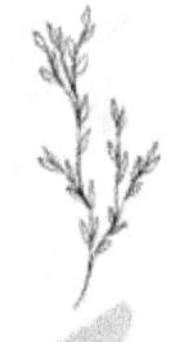

WEEK: MONTH: YEAR:

MONDAY	TUESDAY	WEDNESDAY

THURSDAY	FRIDAY	WEEKEND

NOTES

Daily Meal Planner

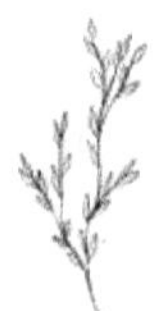

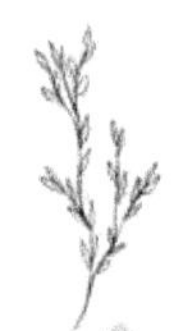

WEEK :   MONTH :   YEAR :

MONDAY	TUESDAY	WEDNESDAY

THURSDAY	FRIDAY	WEEKEND

NOTES

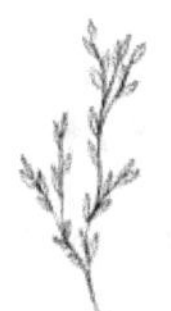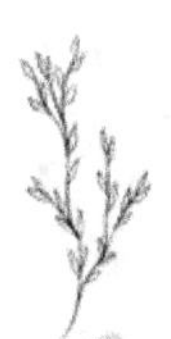

Daily Meal Planner

WEEK : **MONTH :** **YEAR :**

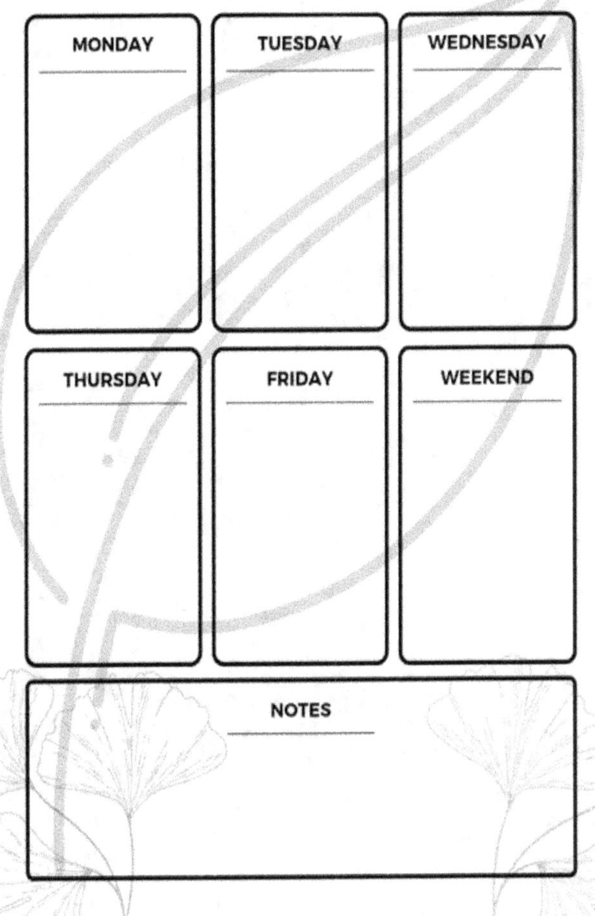

MONDAY	TUESDAY	WEDNESDAY

THURSDAY	FRIDAY	WEEKEND

NOTES

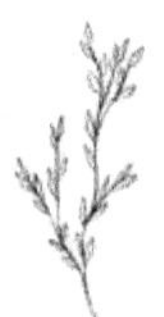

Daily Meal Planner

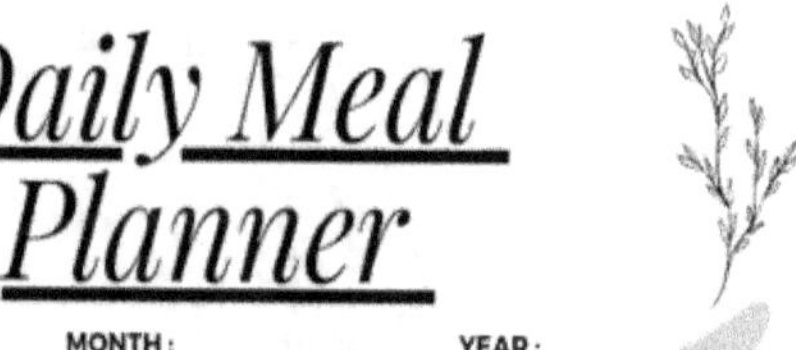

WEEK :   MONTH :   YEAR :

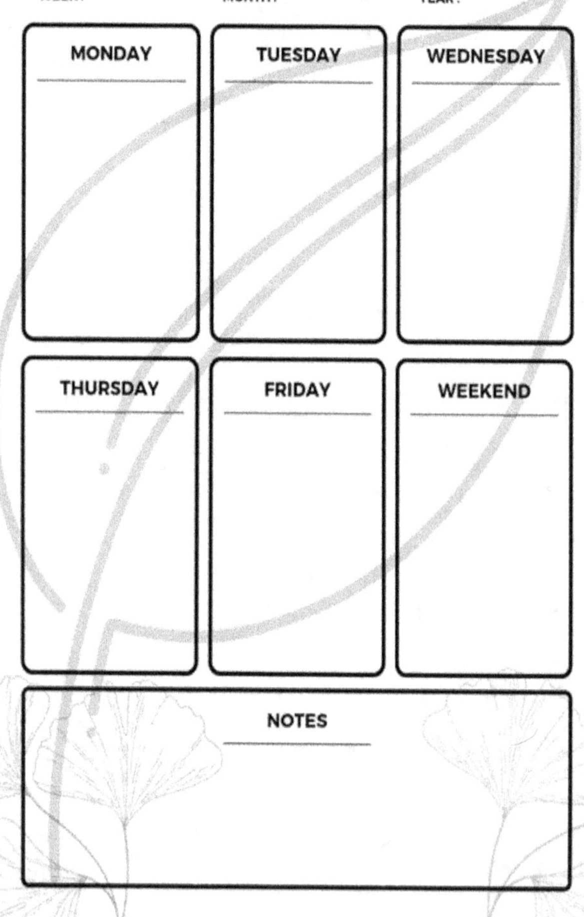

MONDAY

TUESDAY

WEDNESDAY

THURSDAY

FRIDAY

WEEKEND

NOTES

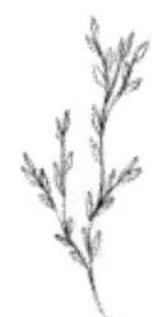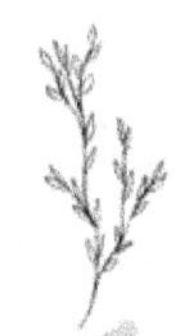

Daily Meal Planner

WEEK: MONTH: YEAR:

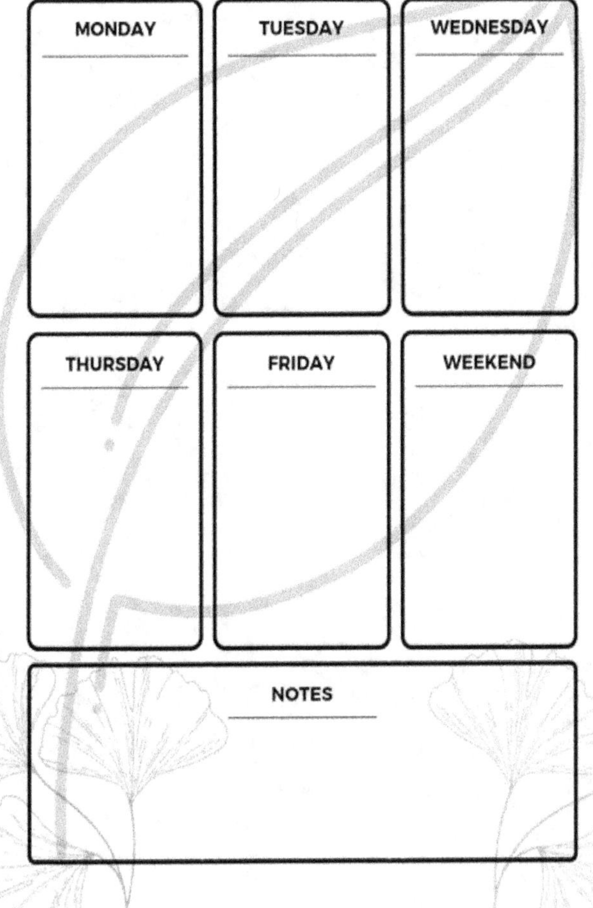

MONDAY	TUESDAY	WEDNESDAY

THURSDAY	FRIDAY	WEEKEND

NOTES

Daily Meal Planner

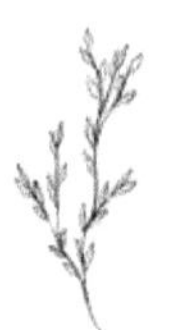 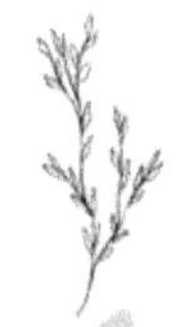

WEEK: MONTH: YEAR:

MONDAY	TUESDAY	WEDNESDAY

THURSDAY	FRIDAY	WEEKEND

NOTES